Basic Electrocardiography
ECG

Stephen Scheidt, MD

Professor of Clinical Medicine
Department of Medicine, Division of Cardiology
Assistant Dean for Continuing Medical Education
The New York Hospital–Cornell Medical Center
New York, New York

with a contribution by
Jay A. Erlebacher, MD

Assistant Professor of Clinical Medicine
The New York Hospital–Cornell Medical Center
New York, New York
Attending Physician, Englewood Hospital
and Holy Name Hospital, Teaneck
New Jersey

illustrated by
Frank H. Netter, MD

CIBA–GEIGY

To
Andrea, Vivian, and Leslie

This volume is adapted from CLINICAL SYMPOSIA, Volume 35,
Number 2, 1983, and Volume 36, Number 6, 1984, both by
Stephen Scheidt, MD, illustrated by Frank H. Netter, MD,
and edited by Werner Heidel, MD

ISBN 0-914168-13-4
Library of Congress Catalog No: 86-63396

Printed in the United States of America

First Printing—1986

Contents

Introduction

The electrocardiogram (ECG) is an indispensable part of medicine. It is routinely performed on almost every hospitalized adult and universally accepted as a simple but highly useful test, even in this age of complex and expensive technology.

Most physicians have had some experience in electrocardiography, but those who do not routinely interpret ECGs may feel somewhat uneasy about their ability in this respect. Textbooks of electrocardiography are often lengthy and detailed and are not intended for brief review. This volume is designed as a concise, practical overview of the subject.

Following a brief consideration of the theoretical basis of electrocardiography, a systematic approach to interpreting the ECG is presented. The sections are arranged to follow the routine of the experienced electrocardiographer, and cover determination of the heart rate, measurement of intervals, derivation of the electrical axis, normal and abnormal cardiac rhythms, atrial and ventricular enlargement or hypertrophy, intraventricular conduction defects (bundle branch and fascicular blocks), myocardial infarction and ischemia, and assessment of ST segment and T wave abnormalities. A brief section covers electrocardiographic manifestations of common artificial cardiac pacemakers. The Atlas of ECG tracings that concludes the volume is keyed to the preceding text, so that the reader can refer to real-life examples of normal and abnormal ECGs.

The last several decades have provided the physician with many new tools for assessing cardiac abnormalities. For example, the echocardiogram is superb in the diagnosis of atrial and ventricular enlargement or hypertrophy, pericardial effusion, and ventricular aneurysm. The stress test and the thallium perfusion scan or gated blood pool radionuclide image are excellent in the diagnosis of myocardial infarction or ischemia. Electrophysiologic studies document conduction abnormalities and assist in the diagnosis and treatment of arrhythmias, while cardiac catheterization is the "gold standard" in the diagnosis of coronary artery disease and valvular and myocardial abnormalities.

Notwithstanding the availability of these and other sophisticated tests, the standard 12-lead ECG can be obtained simply, rapidly, and inexpensively—noninvasive and painless, it poses no risk to the patient. Not only can it be read immediately by trained personnel, it can also be transmitted over continents and interpreted, stored, and retrieved almost instantaneously by computers. Basic ECG interpretation is not immensely difficult, and this volume should inspire and inform those who wish to acquire or improve skills in interpreting ECGs.

Acknowledgments

To my wife, Andrea, and my children, Leslie and Vivian, who have cheerfully tolerated the time I have not spent with them. To my mentors, John H. Laragh and Thomas Killip, III, and my dean, Thomas H. Meikle, Jr, who have been always supportive of teaching and research. To my colleagues, particularly Paul Kligfield and Joseph Hayes, who have taught me much and provided several of the ECGs included herein. And to my patients SZ, AA, DD, SD, and many, many others, who have fulfilled my dream of patients as friends and friends as patients—and whose well-being is the ultimate goal of everything we do.

Basic
Electrocardiography
ECG

THEORETICAL BASIS OF ELECTROCARDIOGRAPHY

Electrical potentials produced by the heart are the sum of minute amounts of the electricity generated from individual cardiac muscle cells. Although electrical potentials generated by the human heart had been recorded a few years earlier, the first crude ECG was reported in 1903 by Willem Einthoven, who used a string galvanometer. Many of the conventions established by Einthoven and other early electrocardiographers still stand and are the basis for much of the format of the modern ECG.

When a string galvanometer was used, an electrical current passed through electrodes connected to two extremities caused deflection of the recording instrument. Passage of current toward the positive end of a bipolar electrode was set to cause a positive deflection of the recorder, which corresponds to an upward movement of the stylus on the standard modern electrocardiograph. Conversely, passage of current away from the positive pole of a bipolar electrode caused a negative deflection, the equivalent of a downward movement of the stylus on today's electrocardiograph. Current flowing at an oblique angle to the electrode caused a smaller deflection of the recorder; the current flowing perpendicular to the electrode did not cause any deflection in the recording instrument attached to that electrode. Einthoven placed various bipolar electrodes, or recording leads, so that it was possible to examine the electrical activity of the heart from several different vantage points.

Plate 1 describes the effects of current flow on ECG deflections according to the respective orientations of the recording lead and the current flow. Consider the lead that is directed horizontally from left to right across the printed page (or from the right arm to the left arm across the chest when one is facing a patient). Electrical current flowing in the same direction as the ECG lead produces the strongest deflection in that lead, which, by convention and by connections within the ECG machine, is arranged to produce a strong upward deflection from the baseline in that lead.

The second panel of Plate 1 represents current flowing generally in the direction of the recording lead, but at a 45° angle. In this case, the oblique vector may be divided into two vectors: a portion parallel to the ECG lead and a portion directed superiorly or inferiorly. Only the portion of the oblique vector that is parallel to the recording lead produces a deflection in the lead. The more closely the direction of the current approximates the direction of the recording lead, the greater is the upward deflection; the more oblique the electrical current, the less strong is the upward deflection in the recording lead.

In the third panel of Plate 1, with current flowing perpendicular to the lead, no current is directed toward the positive end of the recording lead, and thus no ECG deflection occurs in that lead (or upward and downward deflections may be balanced, with a net of zero).

Current flowing directly toward the negative pole of an ECG lead (Plate 1, fourth panel) produces a strong negative deflection in that lead. Current flowing obliquely away from the positive pole, or toward the negative pole, produces a less strong negative deflection, varying according to how closely

Plate 1

Relationship of Current Flow (Depolarization and Repolarization Vectors) to Lead Axis and Consequent Electrocardiographic Deflection

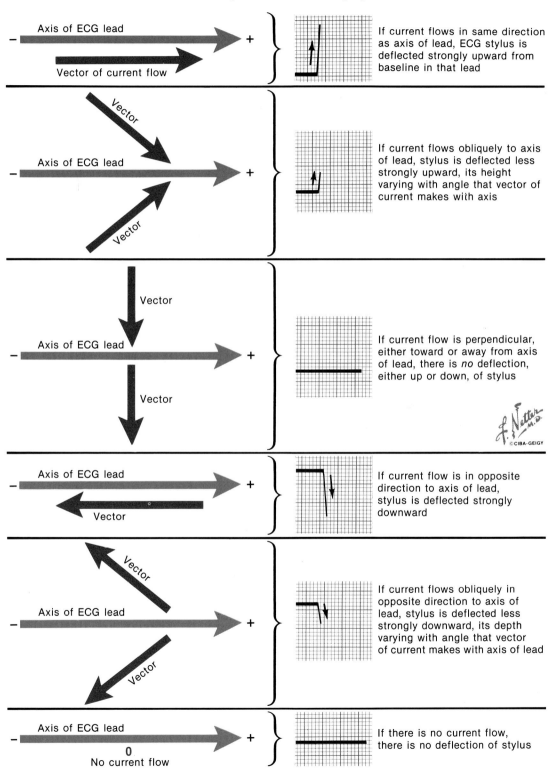

If current flows in same direction as axis of lead, ECG stylus is deflected strongly upward from baseline in that lead

If current flows obliquely to axis of lead, stylus is deflected less strongly upward, its height varying with angle that vector of current makes with axis

If current flow is perpendicular, either toward or away from axis of lead, there is *no* deflection, either up or down, of stylus

If current flow is in opposite direction to axis of lead, stylus is deflected strongly downward

If current flows obliquely in opposite direction to axis of lead, stylus is deflected less strongly downward, its depth varying with angle that vector of current makes with axis of lead

If there is no current flow, there is no deflection of stylus

the current vector is directed toward the axis of the recording lead (Plate 1, fifth panel). If there is no flow of current (Plate 1, last panel), the ECG stylus is not deflected.

The standard limb leads are bipolar electrodes, which were introduced by Einthoven. Although we usually attach electrodes to each of the patient's limbs and may also attach one or more chest leads before recording the ECG, the ECG machine internally switches from one electrode set to another, either automatically or in response to the lead selector switch, so that each designated ECG lead records from only one set of electrodes at a time.

Lead I records the potential between the left arm electrode (arbitrarily designated by Einthoven as the positive pole) and the right arm electrode. Thus, when electrical current moves through the heart from the right arm toward the left arm, a positive deflection is registered in lead I of the ECG (Plate 2, top left). When the ECG selector switch is switched to lead II, a connection is made between the left leg (arbitrarily designated as the positive pole) and the right arm. An electrical current moving from the right arm diagonally downward toward the left leg causes an upward deflection in lead II (Plate 2, top center). The positive pole of lead III is at the left leg and the negative pole at the left arm (Plate 2, top right). Although electrodes are attached to both legs, the right leg electrode is used as a spare or ground, since recordings obtained from either leg electrode are essentially identical.

Leads aVR, aVL and aVF are the augmented limb leads. Originally, these unipolar extremity leads had a common negative pole at zero potential arranged by connecting all four limb leads together within the electrocardiograph. Later, it was discovered that the amplitude of the deflections in these new leads could be increased by disconnecting, within the ECG console, that ground lead attached to the limb being recorded. Thus, the positive pole of the augmented limb leads is at the right arm (lead aVR), the left arm (lead aVL), or the leg (lead aVF). The other two limb leads that are not used as the positive pole become the negative pole, or ground. Plate 2 shows the connections of lead aVR in the center panel, left; of lead aVL in the center panel, middle; and of lead aVF in the center panel, right.

All the leads mentioned thus far are in one plane — the frontal plane. If their vectors are superimposed on a single diagram, these six leads encompass an entire 360° circle (see Plate 8). By convention, the direction toward the left arm is taken as 0°, and radial coordinates are positive reading clockwise and negative reading counterclockwise from the 0° mark. As seen in Plate 8, leads I, II and III point toward 0°, 60°, and 120°, respectively. Lead aVR points toward −150° (the right shoulder), lead aVL is directed toward −30° (the left shoulder), and lead aVF is directed downward at +90° (toward the feet); these leads are not shown in Plate 8 for the sake of clarity.

Several decades after the development of the first electrocardiograph, the need to examine cardiac events in more than one plane became apparent. The precordial leads, introduced into clinical medicine in the 1930s, examine cardiac electrical activity in the horizontal plane, the plane that results if a section is taken from front to back or from sternum to vertebral column (Plate 2, lower left). The negative pole of all precordial electrodes is a common ground arranged within the electrocardiograph by connecting all limb

Plate 2

Electrocardiographic Leads and Their Axes

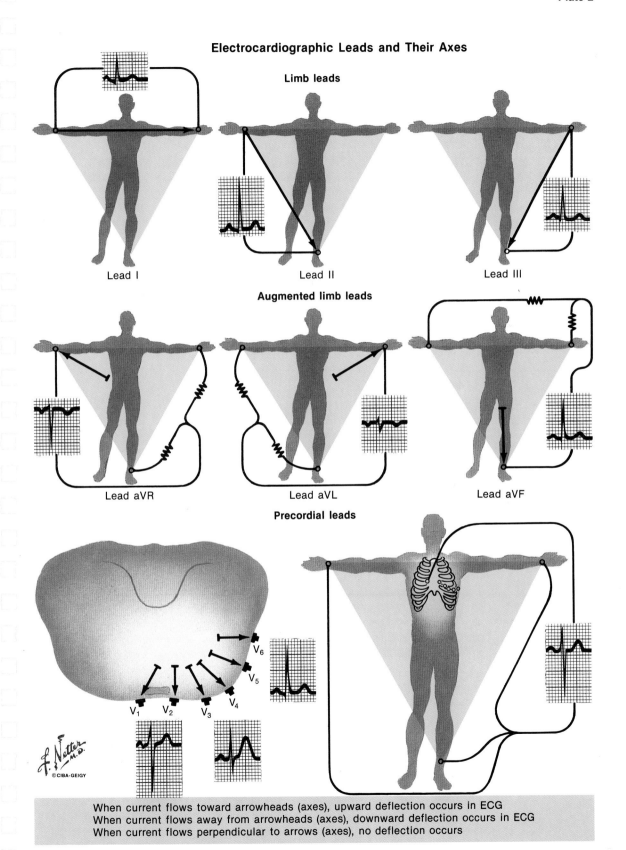

Limb leads

Lead I   Lead II   Lead III

Augmented limb leads

Lead aVR   Lead aVL   Lead aVF

Precordial leads

V_1 V_2 V_3 V_4 V_5 V_6

When current flows toward arrowheads (axes), upward deflection occurs in ECG
When current flows away from arrowheads (axes), downward deflection occurs in ECG
When current flows perpendicular to arrows (axes), no deflection occurs

leads together. The positive poles are placed at the familiar precordial lead positions V_1 through V_6, depicted on the anterior chest in Plate 2, bottom right. In the cross section of the horizontal plane, the vectors represented by these leads are shown in Plate 2, bottom left.

Every reader knows (but it still bears repeating) that all 12 ECG leads described here and others that are not described, such as intracardiac leads, record exactly the same electrical events within the heart. The different positions and orientations of the leads provide varying observation points, and thus the same electrical events may have a different appearance in different leads.

2 NORMAL SEQUENCE OF CARDIAC DEPOLARIZATION AND REPOLARIZATION

The muscle cells of the heart form a syncytium; that is, they are so joined that electrical activity can easily spread from one cell to the next. Actually, spread of electrical activation through the heart is not quite so simple, since certain groups of cardiac cells are designed to rapidly transmit electrical activity through the heart. These specialized cells include the atrial conduction tracts, the atrioventricular (AV) node, the bundle of His, the bundle branches, and the distal ventricular conduction system.

In the resting state, cardiac muscle cells are "polarized," the interior of cells being negatively charged with respect to the exterior. These resting potentials are caused by ionic gradients across the cell membrane; the concentration of potassium ions is much higher inside cells and that of sodium ions is much higher outside. In response to various stimuli, movements of ions occur — particularly a rapid inward movement of sodium, which causes the rapid loss of the internal negative potential. This process is known as "depolarization."

So-called automatic cells in many areas of the heart are capable of spontaneous depolarization and are important in the genesis of some cardiac arrhythmias. However, since the cells of the heart are linked so closely to one another, depolarization beginning in any one area spreads rapidly throughout the entire heart. Under normal conditions, the area that depolarizes most rapidly and thus sets the heart rate is the sinoatrial (SA or sinus) node, a small structure about the size of the period at the end of this sentence, located at the junction of the superior vena cava and the upper right atrium. The depolarization of the tiny SA node is too weak to be seen on the surface ECG, but its activation is inferred from its effect on the adjacent atrial tissue.

Since the SA node is located at the superior right border of the heart, spread of atrial activation from a sinus source is generally downward and somewhat to the left. The atria are rather thin-walled structures with little muscular mass; thus, relatively little electrical activity results from their depolarization. The external recording of normal atrial electrical activity was arbitrarily termed a *P wave* in the early days of electrocardiography. (The beginning letters of the alphabet were probably not used because prior recordings of arterial and venous pulse waves had used "A" and other letters at the beginning of the alphabet for hemodynamic rather than electrocardiographic events.) Plate 3 illustrates the normal sequence of electrical events within the heart and correlates these events with the ECG. Leads I and aVF are used as examples, although any lead could have served for illustration.

As just described, the net electrical vector of all the atrial muscle cells, downward and to the left, is generally toward the positive ends of both leads I and aVF, but the total amount of electrical activity is not particularly large because of the small muscle mass of the atria. Therefore, a small upright deflection is recorded as the initial portion of the ECG in both leads I and aVF — the *P wave* (Plate 3, top).

Once the wave of depolarization reaches the AV node, there is a delay. During this time, electrical activity moves very slowly from the atrium into and through the AV node and then into the proximal portions of the ventricular conduction system, the common bundle of His, and the bundle branches. All these structures are so small that electrical activity within them is not generally detected on the surface ECG, and thus no movement of the baseline is seen — the isoelectric PR interval. (Transvenous electrode catheters passed to the right side of the heart and placed close to the AV node and bundle of His can easily record electrical activation of these structures and have created the new discipline of intracardiac electrophysiology.)

Under normal circumstances, once the wave of depolarization has moved through the AV node, the His bundle, and the early portions of the bundle branches, the first part of the ventricular myocardium to be depolarized is the interventricular septum, from left to right. The initial portion of ventricular depolarization on the surface ECG stems from this septal depolarization. The septum is generally smaller than the great bulk of the ventricular myocardium, and thus this initial deflection is relatively small. Since depolarization is from left to right and slightly downward, this portion of the electrical activation is moving away from the positive end of lead I and produces a small negative deflection in that lead, which early electrocardiographers named a *Q wave*. Since that same septal depolarization is generally downward toward the positive pole of aVF, a small positive deflection is recorded initially in lead aVF (Plate 3, bottom).

Depolarization then spreads along the ventricular conduction system (the distal bundle branches and Purkinje fibers), generally in a predictable fashion: first the septum, next the apex, and then the bulk of the left and right ventricular free walls. In a normal heart, the left ventricle is about 10 mm thick, compared with a maximum of 3 mm for the right ventricle. With depolarization of both ventricles normally occurring at about the same time, the greater muscle mass of the left ventricle generates substantially more electrical activity, and thus the net electrical forces are directed toward it, that is, downward and somewhat to the left. These forces are generally toward the positive end of lead I, and because the muscle mass is so substantial, the electrical potential is also substantial. This produces a large positive or upward deflection in lead I and usually the same in lead aVF, the *R wave* (Plate 4, top).

Ventricular depolarization continues through the remainder of both ventricles; the last area activated is the most superior portion of the left

Plate 3

Normal Sequence of Cardiac Depolarization and Repolarization and Derivation of ECG

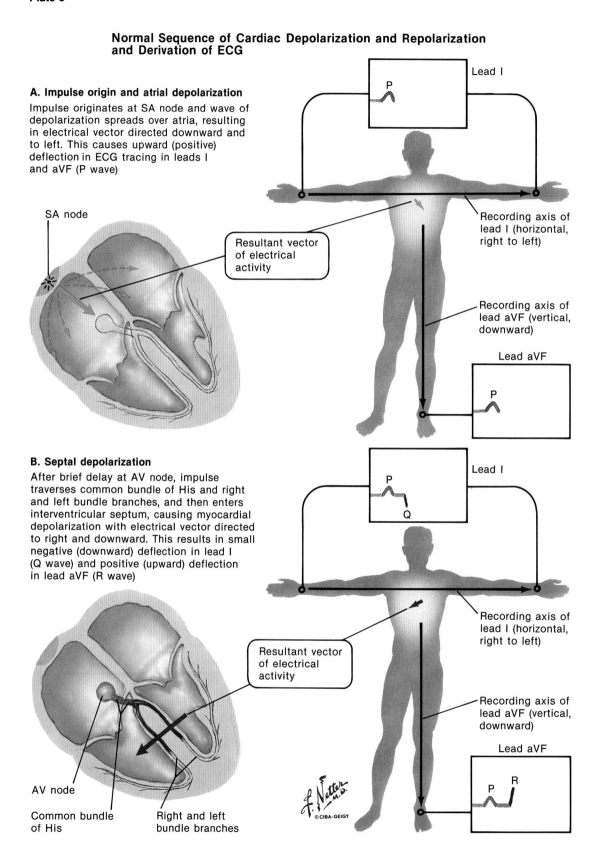

A. Impulse origin and atrial depolarization

Impulse originates at SA node and wave of depolarization spreads over atria, resulting in electrical vector directed downward and to left. This causes upward (positive) deflection in ECG tracing in leads I and aVF (P wave)

SA node

Resultant vector of electrical activity

Lead I

P

Recording axis of lead I (horizontal, right to left)

Recording axis of lead aVF (vertical, downward)

Lead aVF

P

B. Septal depolarization

After brief delay at AV node, impulse traverses common bundle of His and right and left bundle branches, and then enters interventricular septum, causing myocardial depolarization with electrical vector directed to right and downward. This results in small negative (downward) deflection in lead I (Q wave) and positive (upward) deflection in lead aVF (R wave)

Lead I

P

Q

Recording axis of lead I (horizontal, right to left)

Resultant vector of electrical activity

Recording axis of lead aVF (vertical, downward)

Lead aVF

P   R

AV node

Common bundle of His

Right and left bundle branches

Plate 4

Normal Sequence of Cardiac Depolarization and Repolarization and Derivation of ECG (continued)

C. Apical and early ventricular depolarization

Impulse continues along conduction system, causing depolarization of apical ventricular myocardium with electrical vector directed downward and to left. This results in large positive (upward) deflection (R wave) in lead I and extends R wave in lead aVF

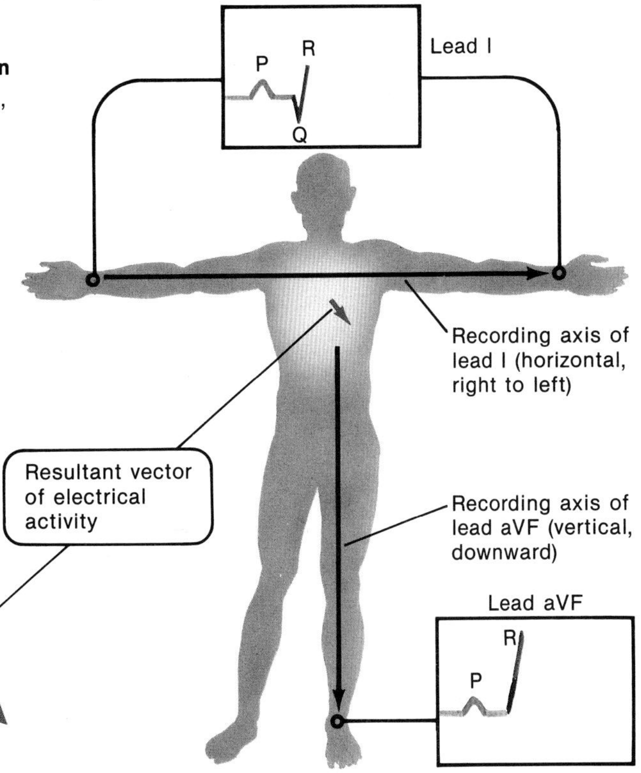

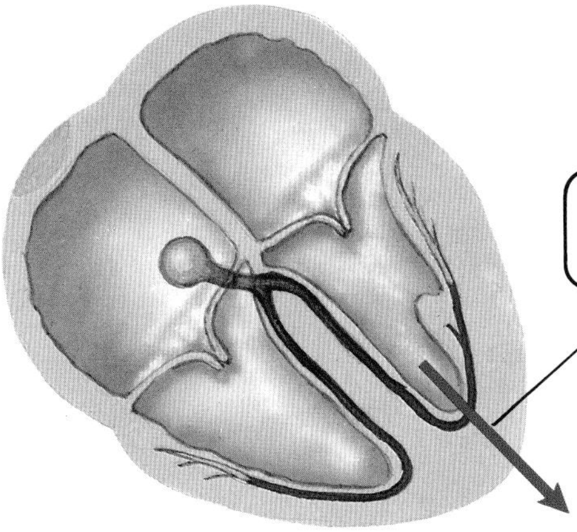

P R Q Lead I

Recording axis of lead I (horizontal, right to left)

Resultant vector of electrical activity

Recording axis of lead aVF (vertical, downward)

Lead aVF

R P

D. Late ventricular depolarization

As depolarization progresses over ventricles, vector shifts to become directed superiorly as well as to left, thus extending upward R wave in lead I and causing negative (downward) deflection (S wave) in lead aVF

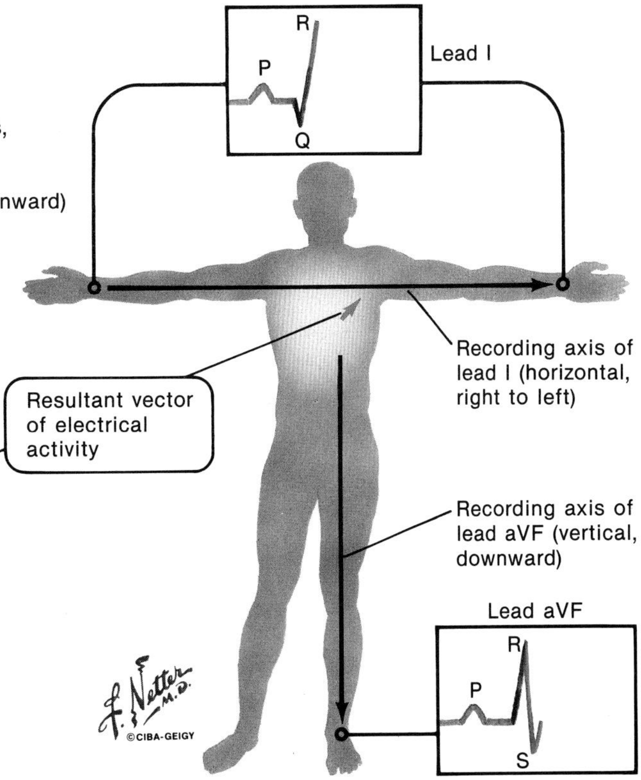

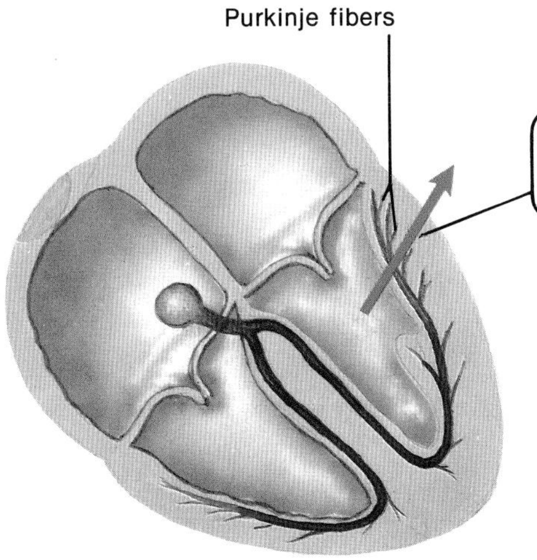

R P Q Lead I

Purkinje fibers

Resultant vector of electrical activity

Recording axis of lead I (horizontal, right to left)

Recording axis of lead aVF (vertical, downward)

Lead aVF

R P S

Plate 5

Normal Sequence of Cardiac Depolarization and Repolarization and Derivation of ECG (continued)

E. Repolarization

When heart is fully depolarized, there is no electrical activity for brief period (ST segment). Then repolarization begins from endocardium to epicardium, producing electrical vector directed downward and to left, causing upward (positive) deflection in both leads I and aVF (T waves). A period of no electrical activity follows, with tracing at baseline until next impulse originates at SA node

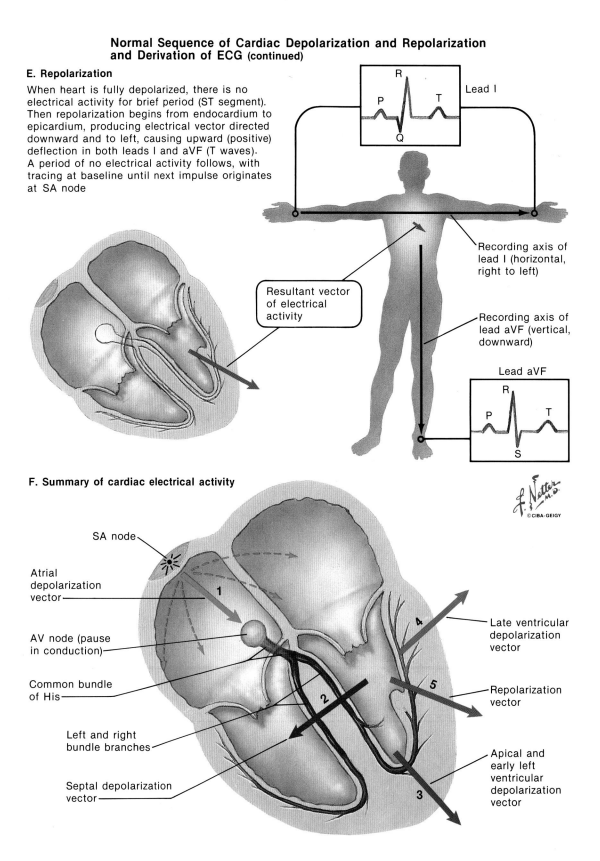

Lead I

Recording axis of lead I (horizontal, right to left)

Recording axis of lead aVF (vertical, downward)

Lead aVF

Resultant vector of electrical activity

F. Summary of cardiac electrical activity

SA node

Atrial depolarization vector

AV node (pause in conduction)

Common bundle of His

Left and right bundle branches

Septal depolarization vector

Late ventricular depolarization vector

Repolarization vector

Apical and early left ventricular depolarization vector

ventricular free wall or the right ventricular outflow tract. By this time, the electrical activity is proceeding generally in a direction opposite to the feet, and thus a negative deflection in lead aVF — the S *wave* — is recorded (Plate 4, bottom). Depending on the bulk of muscle tissue on the high lateral wall of the left ventricle, this vector may or may not cause a terminal negative deflection (S wave) in lead I.

After the ventricle has been totally depolarized, there is little activity until repolarization begins. Thus, the ECG becomes isoelectric for an interval — the *ST segment*. Repolarization, that is, the return of myocardial cells to their resting negative potential, then proceeds from endocardium to epicardium. Again, since the left ventricle is larger than the right ventricle or the atria, its forces are more important in determining the net electrical vector of repolarization, which, in the normal heart, tends to be to the left and downward in the direction of the main muscle mass of the left ventricle. Ventricular repolarization produces the *T wave* (Plate 5, top).

After the conclusion of repolarization, there is again a period of electrical inactivity, and the baseline of the ECG therefore remains isoelectric until the next impulse originates, normally at the SA node, producing the next series of P-QRS-T complexes. The entire sequence of cardiac electrical activity is summarized in Plate 5, bottom.

3 DETERMINATION OF HEART RATE AND ELECTROCARDIOGRAPHIC INTERVALS

Heart Rate

Since ECG paper routinely moves through the machine at a constant speed of 25 mm/second, the horizontal axis on paper represents time. Horizontal lines on standard ECG paper are ruled every millimeter, with darker lines every 5 mm. Five large boxes of 5 mm each equal 25 mm, or 1 second of time. Thus, a single large box 5 mm wide represents 0.20 second, and a single small box 1 mm wide is one-fifth of that, or 0.04 second.

The vertical axis on ECG paper represents voltage. Each ECG machine must be calibrated so that a 1-mv standardization signal produces a deflection of exactly 10 mm (and the standardization should be checked and recorded before every ECG is taken). Thus, each small box of 1 mm in the vertical direction represents 0.10 mv, one large vertical box represents 0.50 mv, and two large vertical boxes represent 1 mv.

Regular heart rates can easily be estimated by measuring the interval between two adjacent complexes. This method of estimating rate can be used for P waves to determine atrial rate, for QRS complexes to determine ventricular rate, for pacemaker spikes to determine pacemaker rate, or for any other regularly occurring event on the ECG. For purposes of simplicity, this discussion refers only to QRS complexes and the determination of ventricular rate.

In Plate 6, the top rhythm strip shows a very rapid ventricular rate with QRS complexes occurring exactly once per large box. Since a large box represents 0.20 second, and there are thus five large boxes in 1 second, it is

Plate 6

Determination of Heart Rate

Regular rhythms

Measure interval between adjacent complexes and relate to large boxes ruled on ECG paper (1 large box represents 0.2 second; thus, there are 300 large boxes/minute)

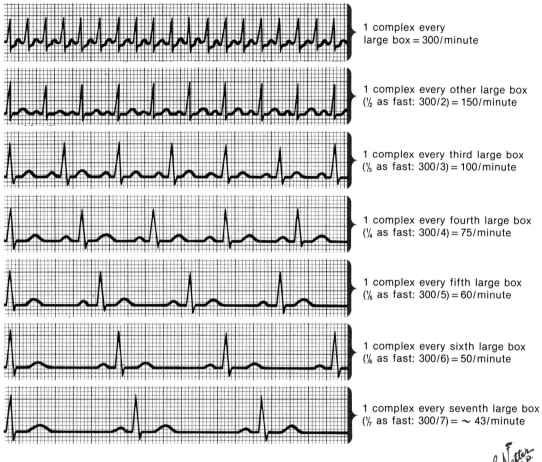

1 complex every large box = 300/minute

1 complex every other large box (½ as fast: 300/2) = 150/minute

1 complex every third large box (⅓ as fast: 300/3) = 100/minute

1 complex every fourth large box (¼ as fast: 300/4) = 75/minute

1 complex every fifth large box (⅕ as fast: 300/5) = 60/minute

1 complex every sixth large box (⅙ as fast: 300/6) = 50/minute

1 complex every seventh large box (⅐ as fast: 300/7) = ~ 43/minute

Irregular rhythms

Count number of complexes over given period of time, usually in 6-second interval included within 2 time markers at top border of ECG paper

|← Marks every 15 large boxes (3 seconds) →|←—————— 3 seconds ——————→|

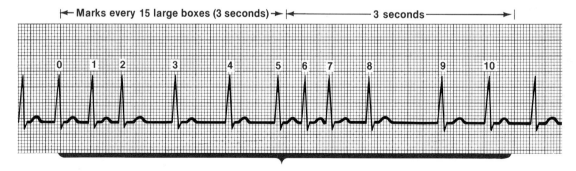

Find complex that coincides with time marker at top. Then count number of complexes in span of 30 large boxes, i.e., 2 groups of 15 boxes each as marked by lines or dots at top of ECG paper (in this case, 10½). Since each large box = 0.2 second, 30 large boxes = 30 x 0.2 = 6 seconds. Multiply by 10 to give rate/60 seconds (in this case, 10½ x 10 = rate of 105/minute)

clear that there are 60 × 5, or 300, large boxes in 1 minute. Any reader who doubts this and who has considerable patience, may mark a strip of ECG paper, start the paper running at the usual speed of 25 mm/second, and count boxes exactly 1 minute later; 300 large boxes will have passed a given point in 1 minute. Thus, if a QRS complex occurs once with every large box, the QRS rate must be 300/minute.

In the second rhythm strip in Plate 6, QRS complexes occur with every second large box. It is unimportant that the tip of the QRS complex does not actually occur on one of the heavy vertical lines; if ECG calipers are placed between the peaks or between any similar points of two adjacent ECG complexes and then moved over to a heavy vertical line, it is easily seen that the QRS complexes occur regularly with every second large box. Since large boxes occur 300 times/minute, a QRS complex occurring with every second box must have a rate of 300 divided by 2, or 150/minute. In the third strip in Plate 6, QRS complexes are occurring with every third large box; the rate must be one-third of 300, or 100/minute. Similarly, QRS complexes occurring every fourth large box have a rate of 300 divided by 4, or 75/minute; complexes occurring every fifth large box have a rate of 300 divided by 5, or 60/minute; complexes occurring every sixth large box have a rate of 300 divided by 6, or 50/minute, and so forth.

What if the QRS rate is regular, but ECG complexes do not occur precisely with a whole number of large boxes? Examine, for example, the top rhythm strip in Plate 10, in which QRS complexes occur a bit less often than every fourth box, which would be a rate of 300 divided by 4, or 75/minute, but significantly more often than every fifth box, which would represent a rate of 300 divided by 5, or 60/minute. The rate must be less than 75 but more than 60/minute. In this case, the interval between adjacent QRS complexes is considerably closer to four than to five boxes, and thus the ventricular rate will be considerably closer to 75 than 60. For this strip, one would estimate a rate a bit below 75, perhaps 72. In point of fact, the exact heart rate is 71.4/minute. Practically speaking, an estimate within 5 beats per minute or so is more than satisfactory for almost all clinical purposes, except the evaluation of artificial pacemakers, and thus the experienced electrocardiographer can "eyeball" regular cardiac rhythms and give satisfactory estimates of the actual rate by extrapolation without measurement.

For irregular rhythms, any method of rate calculation that depends on intervals between complexes is unreliable, since these intervals are constantly changing. With irregular rhythms such as atrial fibrillation, it is necessary to actually count the number of complexes over a period of time. Most ECG paper has markings at the top or bottom margin, as shown in the rhythm strip in the bottom portion of Plate 6. Although different manufacturers use different types of markings, a vertical ruled line or dot is common, and these are generally spaced 15 large boxes (or 15 × 0.2 = 3.0 seconds) apart.

Most electrocardiographers count the number of complexes occurring in two of these 3-second periods; that is, they count complexes falling in a 6-second period and then multiply by 10 to give the heart rate/60 seconds. In the example shown in Plate 6, bottom, the ECG strip is scanned until a complex is found that falls exactly on one of the 3-second marker lines. This complex is the zero complex, not the first complex. Then the number of QRS complexes is counted, as in the example, up to the end of the 6-second period. In the example shown, there are 10 complexes, and part of the interval toward the eleventh complex. Multiplying the 6-second count of 10 1/2 by 10 gives an estimated ventricular rate of 105/minute.

Electrocardiographic Intervals

After determination of the heart rate, several important electrocardiographic intervals are considered, as depicted in Plate 7, top. These intervals are usually measured with calipers. The electrocardiographer places the calipers at the beginning and end of the wave or interval under consideration and then shifts over to the ruled lines for ease of estimation, bearing in mind that each small horizontal box represents 0.04 second and each large horizontal box represents 0.04 × 5, or 0.20 second.

The *P wave* begins with the first upward deflection from the baseline and ends with return to the baseline. The normal P wave measures less than 0.11 second in width, or not quite three small boxes.

The *PR interval* is measured from the first upward deflection of the P wave to the first deflection of the QRS from the baseline, whether negative (Q) or positive (R). The normal PR interval varies slightly according to age and heart rate, but for all practical purposes, can be said to range from 0.12 to 0.20 second, or three to five small boxes. (The *PR segment*, although shown in Plate 7, top, is almost never measured.) The *QRS interval* is measured from the first deflection of the QRS from the baseline, whether negative or positive, to the eventual return of the QRS to the baseline. The QRS interval should be less than 0.10 second, or two and one-half small boxes.

The *ST segment* is measured from the return of the QRS to the baseline until the first upward or downward deflection of the T wave. While the duration of the ST segment is not generally of clinical significance, it is an exceedingly important portion of the ECG because of shifts up or down from the baseline, which may be associated with ischemic heart disease, pericarditis, or other conditions. It should be noted that shifts in the ST segment, whether elevations or depressions, are generally measured at a point 0.08 second (80 msec), or two small boxes, after the end of the QRS complex.

The *QT interval* is measured from the beginning of the QRS complex to the final return of the T wave to the baseline. The QT interval is markedly affected by heart rate, and formulas or tables that take heart rate into account must be used to obtain the upper limits of normal. The most common formula used, that of Bazett, derives a corrected QT interval, or QT_c, from the formula $QT_c = QT \div \sqrt{RR\ interval}$. Since it is inconvenient to deal with formulas and square roots, most electrocardiographers consult charts such as that reproduced in Plate 7, bottom.

For the guidance of the beginning ECG reader, one might generalize that with normal heart rates, 60 to 100/minute, QT intervals are generally in the range of 0.30 to 0.40 second, and the maximum QT interval is generally about 10% longer in females than in males. Even the experienced electrocardiographer must consult the chart to be certain, but when QT intervals exceed 0.40 to 0.44 second, the interval is probably abnormally prolonged unless the heart rate is extremely slow.

Plate 7

Electrocardiographic Waves, Intervals, and Segments

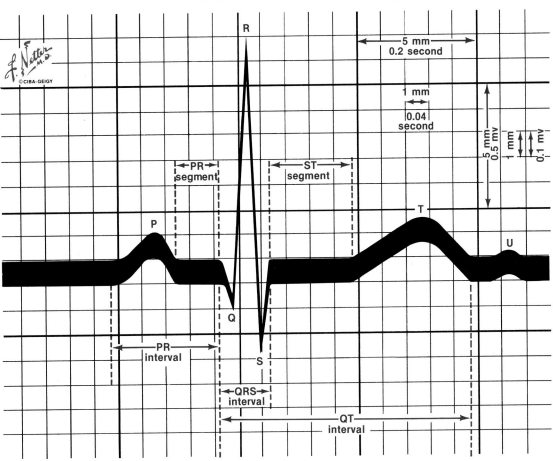

Data for computing heart rate, with maximum QT intervals at various rates

Heart rate	Cycle time (0.04–second intervals)	Maximum QT (seconds)		Heart rate	Cycle time (0.04–second intervals)	Maximum QT (seconds)	
		Male	Female			Male	Female
300	5	.19	.20	68	22	.38	.41
250	6	.20	.22	65	23	.38	.42
214	7	.21	.23	62	24	.39	.43
187	8	.23	.25	60	25	.40	.44
166	9	.24	.26	57	26	.41	.45
150	10	.25	.28	55	27	.42	.46
136	11	.26	.29	52	28	.42	.47
125	12	.28	.30	50	30	.44	.48
115	13	.29	.32	46	32	.45	.50
107	14	.30	.33	43	34	.47	.51
100	15	.31	.34	41	36	.48	.53
93	16	.32	.35	39	38	.49	.54
88	17	.33	.36	37	40	.51	.56
83	18	.34	.37	35	42	.52	.57
78	19	.35	.38	34	44	.53	.58
75	20	.36	.39	32	46	.54	.60
71	21	.37	.40	30	50	.57	.62

The chart in Plate 7, bottom, is also useful for more precise determination of heart rate with regular rhythms. "Cycle time" is just a technical term for the number of small boxes (0.04-second intervals) between two adjacent complexes. As discussed before and shown in Plate 6, adjacent QRS complexes occurring every five small boxes, or once every large box, indicate a heart rate of 300/minute. As previously noted in the discussion on determination of regular heart rates, complexes occurring every second large box, or every 10 small boxes, have a rate of 300 divided by 2, or 150; complexes occurring every third large box, or every 15 small boxes, a rate of 300 divided by 3, or 100, and so on. If QRS complexes are not exactly one, two, three, or some other whole number of large boxes apart, the chart in Plate 7 can be used. For instance, examine Plate 10, top, where adjacent QRS complexes occur not quite four large boxes (or 20 small boxes) apart, but rather every 21 small boxes. A "cycle time" of 21 in the chart in Plate 7 is equal to a heart rate of 71/minute.

4 ELECTRICAL AXIS

Calculation of the direction of electrical activity, or electrical axis, is frequently confusing and often distracts the beginner from much more important findings. Precise calculation of axis is immensely complicated, since the orientation of electrical activity is constantly changing as depolarization and repolarization of various cardiac chambers proceed throughout the electrocardiographic cycle. Plotting of the electrical axis at any given instant can be done by the vectorcardiogram every few milliseconds throughout the cardiac cycle. Although this device may be slightly more accurate than the standard ECG in a few circumstances, it is rarely used because its greater complexity and cost do not seem to be justified in terms of diagnostic yield. With use of the standard ECG, "axis" means the net direction of electrical activity, usually summed over the entire duration of atrial or ventricular activation.

The P wave, or atrial electrical axis, is rarely determined. The T wave, or ventricular repolarization axis, is significant in certain circumstances. For example, the T wave axis often shifts away from an ischemic or infarcted area of myocardium and thus aids in localizing that area. The QRS, or ventricular depolarization axis, though, is most important, and when "axis" alone is discussed, it refers to the QRS axis.

There is a general correlation between the electrical axis of the QRS complex and the anatomy of the heart. Major hypertrophy of either ventricle tends to displace the axis in the direction of the hypertrophied ventricle. Changes in conduction, whether caused by disease of the myocardium or intrinsic disease of the conduction system, also cause axis shifts.

The normal electrical axis of the QRS is from $+90°$ or $+105°$ to $-15°$ or $-30°$. This imprecision may seem strange, but there is no single recognized authority for electrocardiography, and various experts have suggested slightly different limits for the normal electrical axis of the QRS. The area between $+90°$ and $+105°$ is in dispute, but almost all would agree that a QRS axis further right than $+105°$ constitutes *right axis deviation*. Conditions that might cause right axis deviation are chronic obstructive lung disease, pulmonary emboli, certain types of congenital heart disease, and other disorders that cause severe pulmonary hypertension and cor pulmonale (Plate 8, top left).

The area between $-15°$ and $-29°$ is a gray area, on the borderline of left axis deviation, but most authorities would agree that an axis left of $-30°$ constitutes *left axis deviation*. Hypertension, aortic valvular disease, and ischemic heart disease, or other diseases predominantly affecting the left ventricle, as well as certain defects of intraventricular conduction, are among the causes of left axis deviation (Plate 8, top right).

The axis can be calculated exactly by plotting vectors on a triaxial reference grid, which is nothing more than a rearranged Einthoven triangle. The triaxial reference system using standard leads I, II and III is shown in Plate 8, bottom. In the illustration, leads I and III are used and the QRS axis is determined; however, the method applies to calculation of any axis, and any two frontal leads may be used.

First, the algebraic sum of the QRS is determined in millimeters. In lead I, the Q wave is -2.5 mm deep and the R wave is $+16$ mm high, for an algebraic sum of $+13.5$ mm. The point corresponding to $+13.5$ mm is located on lead I, and a perpendicular is dropped from that point. In lead III, the R wave is $+14$ mm high and the S wave is -5 mm deep, for an algebraic sum of $+9$ mm. The point corresponding to $+9$ mm is found on lead III, and the perpendicular is dropped from that point. A line drawn from the center of the triaxial diagram to the intersection of the two perpendiculars gives the electrical axis; in the illustration, it is about $+53°$, which is within the normal range for a QRS axis (shaded area on the diagram).

The triaxial vectorial method of axis determination, although precise, is far too cumbersome for everyday use. Most experienced electrocardiographers use an approximate method in which the axis can be quickly estimated by inspection. The approximate method of axis estimation requires inspection of several leads of the ECG in a particular order (Plate 9). This method depends on the fact that a positive QRS complex in any given lead means the axis is directed toward the positive pole of that lead, while a negative QRS complex means the axis is directed away from the positive pole of the lead.

With this method, first examine lead I. If the QRS is negative, its axis must be directed away from the positive pole of lead I, somewhere in the shaded area of Plate 9, top right. Although the axis might be either to the right of $+90°$ or to the left of $-90°$, both in the shaded area, a QRS axis between $-90°$ and $180°$ rarely if ever occurs. In the case of a negative QRS in lead I, it is much more likely that the axis is directed to the right (clockwise) of $+90°$, or generally in the direction of the right ventricle.

As noted previously, the area between $+90°$ and $+105°$ is in some dispute; most authorities are not certain of right axis deviation unless the axis is to the right of $+105°$; however, with the exception of children and adolescents (who may normally have forces directed a bit more toward the right ventricle), a negative QRS in lead I, denoting an axis to the right of $+90°$, should alert the physician to the possibility of right axis deviation. If the QRS is also positive in lead aVR (not shown on the diagram), right axis

Plate 8

Electrical Axis of Heart

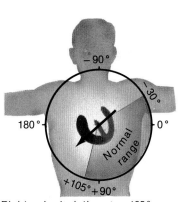

Right axis deviation: ≥ +105°, e.g., chronic obstructive lung disease and pulmonary hypertension

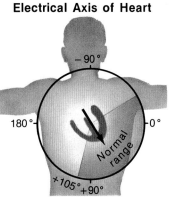

Normal electrical axis: −29° to +105°

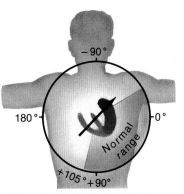

Left axis deviation: ≥ −30° (more negative), e.g., hypertension or aortic stenosis with major left ventricular predominance

Triaxial reference (vectorial) method of axis determination

Sum of QRS in mm in lead I and lead III (or in leads I and II) is determined and plotted on vectorial diagram below

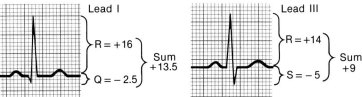

Lead I

R = +16
Q = −2.5
Sum +13.5

Lead III

R = +14
S = −5
Sum +9

Perpendiculars (blue) are drawn at plotted points on respective vectorial reference lines. Line (red) drawn from central point through intersection of perpendiculars gives electrical axis (in this case about +53°, which is within normal range)

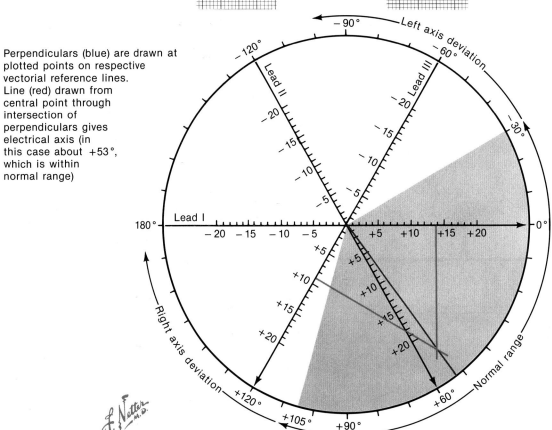

F. Netter M.D.
©CIBA-GEIGY

Plate 9

Practical (Approximate) Method of Electrical Axis Determination

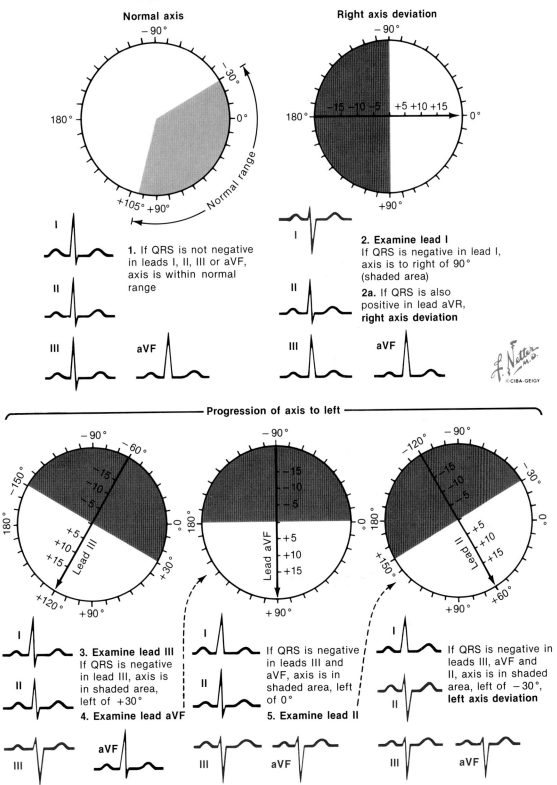

Normal axis

1. If QRS is not negative in leads I, II, III or aVF, axis is within normal range

Right axis deviation

2. **Examine lead I**
If QRS is negative in lead I, axis is to right of 90° (shaded area)

2a. If QRS is also positive in lead aVR, **right axis deviation**

— Progression of axis to left —

3. **Examine lead III**
If QRS is negative in lead III, axis is in shaded area, left of +30°

4. **Examine lead aVF**
If QRS is negative in leads III and aVF, axis is in shaded area, left of 0°

5. **Examine lead II**
If QRS is negative in leads III, aVF and II, axis is in shaded area, left of −30°, **left axis deviation**

deviation is definite. If, as in most patients, the QRS is positive in lead I, right axis deviation is *excluded.*

Next examine lead III. Since the positive pole of lead III is located inferiorly and to the right at +120°, the boundary between positivity and negativity in lead III is the perpendicular to lead III, or a line from +30° to −150°. Again, since a QRS axis in the vicinity of −150° is anatomically almost impossible, a positive QRS in lead III means a QRS axis to the right of +30°, and a negative QRS in lead III means an axis in the shaded area to the left (counterclockwise) of +30°.

Next examine lead aVF (Plate 9, center bottom). The boundary between a positive and a negative QRS in lead aVF is at 0°. A negative QRS in lead aVF is in the shaded area to the left (counterclockwise) of 0°.

Finally, examine lead II. The boundary between a positive and a negative QRS in lead II is at −30°. A negative QRS in lead II means a QRS axis left of −30°, clearly in the area of left axis deviation. By examining leads III, aVF and II in order, one can readily estimate the QRS axis. If a QRS is positive in lead I and positive in leads III, aVF and II, the QRS axis is in the normal range between +90° and +30°. If the QRS is negative in lead III but positive in aVF, the axis must be between +30° and 0° (one may think of moving the shaded area in a counterclockwise direction). If the QRS is negative in leads III and aVF but positive in lead II, the axis must be between 0° and −30°. If the QRS is negative in all three leads — III, aVF and II — the axis is all the way left beyond −30°.

If the algebraic sum of the QRS in any given lead is 0 (the positive deflection exactly equals the negative deflection), the QRS axis must be exactly on the perpendicular to that lead. If the positive deflection does not exactly balance the negative deflection in any lead, the QRS axis can be estimated as being between the perpendiculars of two leads; this generally results in an error of no more than 5° to 10°, which is precise enough for the usual clinical purposes.

In summary, to approximate the electrical axis, one looks for negative QRS complexes and, by so doing, places the QRS axis in the area pointing toward the negative pole of that lead, or the shaded area. A positive QRS in *both* leads I and II means the axis is normal. A negative QRS in lead I means a QRS axis to the right of 90°, and raises the possibility of right axis deviation. The QRS is then examined in turn in leads III, aVF and II. The QRS axis is to the left of +30° if the QRS is negative in lead III; to the left of 0° if the QRS is negative in leads III and aVF; and to the left of −30° (definite left axis deviation) if the QRS is negative in leads III, aVF and II.

5 | DIAGNOSIS OF CARDIAC RHYTHM

Although lengthy textbooks have been written on the subject of cardiac rhythm diagnosis, the vast majority of arrhythmias can be diagnosed by determining the answers to five simple questions.

1. What is the atrial rhythm? (Look for the P waves.)
2. What is the ventricular rhythm? (Look at the QRS complexes.)

3. Is AV conduction normal? (What is the relationship between the P waves and the QRS complexes?)
4. Are there any unusual complexes? (Are there early complexes, late complexes, or complexes of unusual contour?)
5. Is the rhythm dangerous?

Supraventricular Rhythms

To answer the first question — "What is the atrial rhythm?" — the electrocardiographer searches for P waves. In normal sinus rhythm, P waves are easily found in their expected location just preceding the QRS complex. Obviously, in an arrhythmia they may not be in this location, and some searching may be necessary. The following clues may help in finding P waves:

• P waves are usually — although not always — regular. Thus, one looks for small, regular deflections. When the baseline is isoelectric, for example, between the end of a T wave and the beginning of the next QRS complex, P waves should be easy to find, but if P waves occur at the same time as the QRS complex or a T wave, the smaller P wave may be wholly or partially buried in the larger wave.

The experienced electrocardiographer looks for tiny variations in the shape of the QRS complex or the T wave and attempts to relate these to regular occurrences that might be P waves. If two adjacent deflections that appear to be adjacent P waves are found on one portion of a tracing, the electrocardiographer will set calipers to that interval and "march" the interval across the remainder of the tracing to see whether deformations of QRS complexes or T waves betray the presence of P waves wherever calipers indicate that regular P waves should occur.

• Since the right atrium is in the superior right portion of the heart, atrial activation usually — although not always — spreads downward and to the left. Thus, the axis of atrial electrical activity is oriented most directly toward leads II and aVF in the frontal plane and toward lead V_1 in the sagittal plane. These leads, then, tend to have the largest P waves and are the best places to search for P waves if they are not obvious.

A sinus origin is assumed if P waves are regular and upright in leads II, III and aVF (signifying a P wave axis down and toward the left, which implies a P wave origin at the upper right portion of the atrium, the area of the SA node). If the heart rate is 60 to 100/minute, *normal sinus rhythm* is present (Plate 10A). If the rate is less than 60/minute, *sinus bradycardia* is present (Plate 10B, Atlas ECG 5-1). This may be caused by increased vagal or parasympathetic tone or occur in the acute stages of myocardial infarction, particularly diaphragmatic infarction.

If the rate is greater than 100/minute, *sinus tachycardia* is diagnosed (Plate 10C, Atlas ECG 5-2). Sinus tachycardia is most often a physiologic response to exercise, fever, pain, fear, or other stresses, but may also be a clue to occult congestive heart failure or other cardiac decompensation.

If all P waves are identical and upright in leads II, III and aVF, but rhythmically irregular, further measurement is necessary. If the longest PP or RR interval exceeds the shortest such interval by 0.16 second (four small boxes) or more, *sinus arrhythmia* is diagnosed.

Plate 10

Supraventricular Rhythms

A. Normal sinus rhythm

Impulses originate at SA node at normal rate

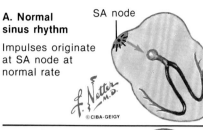

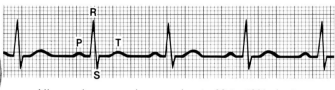

All complexes evenly spaced; rate 60 to 100/minute

B. Sinus bradycardia

Impulses originate at SA node at slow rate

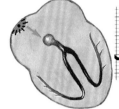

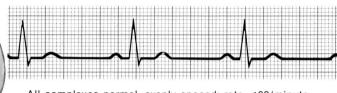

All complexes normal, evenly spaced; rate <60/minute

C. Sinus tachycardia

Impulses originate at SA node at rapid rate

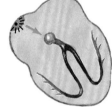

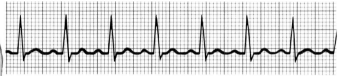

All complexes normal, evenly spaced; rate >100/minute

D. Sinus arrhythmia

Impulses originate at SA node at varying rate

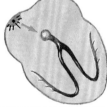

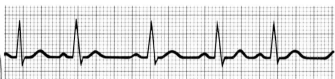

All complexes normal but rhythmically irregular. Longest PP or RR interval exceeds shortest by 0.16 second or more

E. Nonsinus atrial (coronary sinus) rhythm

Impulses originate low in atrium; travel retrograde as well as distally

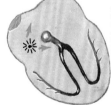

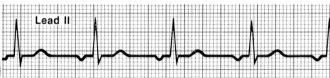

Lead II

P waves inverted in leads II, III and aVF

F. Wandering atrial pacemaker

Impulses originate from varying points in atria

Variation in P wave contour, PR interval, PP and thus RR intervals

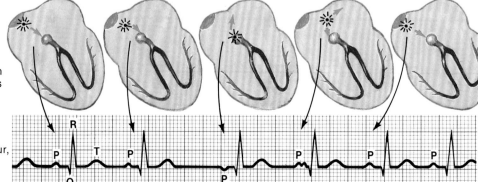

Plate 11

Supraventricular Rhythms (continued)

G. Multifocal atrial tachycardia (MAT)

Impulses originate irregularly and rapidly at different points in atria

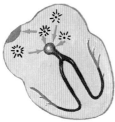

Usually associated with severe pulmonary disease

P wave contours, PR intervals, PP and thus RR intervals all may vary

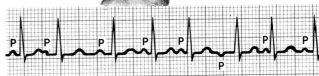

H. Paroxysmal atrial tachycardia (PAT)

Impulses recycle repeatedly in and near AV node due to slowing in area of unidirectional block

4. Repolarization completed, which allows:

5. Recycling impulse

1. α pathway within AV node

3. Shaded area of abnormal conduction stops normal antegrade wave front (unidirectional block) and slows returning impulse

2. β pathway within AV node

Atrial rate 160 to 220/minute. P waves regular and often inverted. QRS regular or irregular

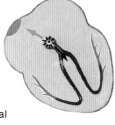

I. Atrial flutter

Impulses travel in circular course in atria, setting up regular, rapid (220 to 300/minute) flutter (F) waves without any isoelectric baseline

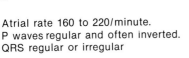

Variable block

Lead II

Rapid flutter (F) waves. Ventricular rate (QRS) regular or irregular and slower (depending on degree of block)

J. Atrial fibrillation

Impulses take chaotic, random pathways in atria

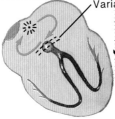

Coarse fibrillation   **Fine fibrillation**

Baseline coarsely or finely irregular; P waves absent. Ventricular response (QRS) irregular, slow or rapid

K. Junctional rhythm

Impulses originate in AV node with retrograde and antegrade transmission

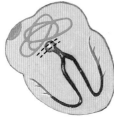

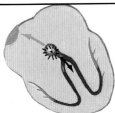

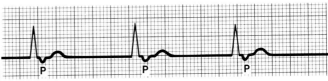

P wave, often inverted, may be buried in QRS or follow QRS. Rate slow, QRS narrow

In the example in Plate 10D, the interval between the first and second P waves is 16 small boxes, or 0.64 second. The interval between the second and third P waves is 21 small boxes, or 0.84 second. The interval between the third and fourth P waves is close to, although slightly less than, the interval between the second and third P waves, whereas the interval between the fourth and fifth P waves is the shortest of all — 15 small boxes (0.60 second). The difference between the longest PP interval (0.84 second) and the shortest PP interval (0.60 second) exceeds 0.16 second, and thus sinus arrhythmia is diagnosed (Atlas ECG 5-3).

Actually, *sinus irregularity* is probably a better term. This rhythm is extremely common, the rule rather than the exception in normal children and young persons; thus, calling it an "arrhythmia" seems misleading. Sinus irregularity in young persons without evidence of heart disease is a normal variant. In the elderly, however, sinus irregularity, as well as sinus bradycardia, sinus pauses, and sinus arrest (page 36), may be signs of degenerative disease of the SA node, usually called "sick sinus syndrome."

If all P waves are identical and regular but inverted in leads II, III and aVF, the P wave axis is highly abnormal, implying an origin other than the SA node located in the upper right corner of the atrium. Some years ago, such rhythms were considered to originate from the coronary sinus, the anatomic structure that empties venous blood from the myocardium into the low right atrium. However, precise intracardiac electrophysiologic studies have shown that many rhythms with an unusual P wave axis do not necessarily originate in the coronary sinus, and thus the old term "coronary sinus rhythm" has been replaced by *nonsinus atrial rhythm* (Plate 10E, Atlas ECG 5-4).

If the contour or shape of P waves varies from beat to beat in a single lead, often associated with variation of the PR interval and the PP and thus RR intervals, it seems likely that the site of atrial depolarization is varying — *wandering atrial pacemaker* (Plate 10F, Atlas ECG 5-5). Both wandering atrial pacemaker and nonsinus atrial rhythm tend to occur in patients whose SA node is not functioning properly for one reason or another. These arrhythmias may also be manifestations of atrial abnormalities, as in rheumatic heart disease.

Multifocal atrial tachycardia (MAT) (Plate 11G, Atlas ECG 5-6) is similar to wandering atrial pacemaker. In MAT, P wave contours, PR intervals, and PP and thus RR intervals all may vary. The differentiation from wandering atrial pacemaker is solely that the rate is much increased in MAT, usually to more than 100/minute, and it is almost invariably associated with severe pulmonary disease (often with respiratory decompensation) or with congestive heart failure.

Paroxysmal atrial tachycardia (PAT) is often a reentry tachycardia. It is characterized by P waves that are regular, identical, frequently inverted in lead II, and very rapid — usually 160 to 220/minute. PAT may occur in patients with rheumatic heart disease, pulmonary disease, or cardiac decompensation. It is common in patients with the Wolff-Parkinson-White syndrome (page 27) and is seen in some patients with mitral valve prolapse or digitalis intoxication. It also may occur in normal persons with no obvious structural heart disease.

The pathogenesis of PAT is generally an area of abnormal conduction. An impulse normally can travel several possible pathways from the atria through the AV node. Two possible routes are often schematically drawn as an α pathway and a β pathway (Plate 11H,1 and 2). Under normal circumstances, depolarization should proceed from the crest of the AV node downward, passing antegrade (from top to bottom) in both α and β pathways in a relatively uniform fashion. Patients with PAT have an area of abnormal conduction (shaded area, Plate 11H,3), which produces unidirectional block; that is, an impulse can proceed in an antegrade direction down the α pathway but is blocked from proceeding down the β pathway. The impulse, having reached the bottom of the AV node via the α pathway, is then able to return to its starting point via the β pathway.

The impulse travels in a retrograde direction but is slowed by the area of abnormal conduction. By the time it reaches the starting point at the crest of the AV node, depolarization and repolarization have been completed, and cells at that point are capable of being reexcited by the returning impulse. The impulse then starts down again or "reenters" its original pathway before the SA node is ready with the next normal impulse, and the cycle is repeated over and over again in rapid succession, producing a so-called reentry tachycardia. Discrete P waves are seen on the ECG, and if other complexes do not interfere, one may see areas of isoelectric baseline between P waves (Atlas ECGs 5-7 and 5-8).

In contradistinction, in *atrial flutter*, the baseline is never isoelectric. Flutter is characterized by rapid, identical undulating waves that are of longer duration and sometimes of considerably greater amplitude than P waves. Indeed, they are so unlike P waves that they are usually called F or "flutter" waves (Plate 11I, Atlas ECG 5-9). Instead of the anatomically small reentry pathway confined to the AV node and environs that is characteristic of PAT, flutter impulses may travel in a rather large, generally circular course within the atria and produce larger and continuous F waves. These F waves often have a rate close to 300/minute; some degree of AV block is usually present. If AV block is regular at 2:1, 3:1, or 4:1, and so forth, the QRS rate will be some exact fraction of 300, often exactly 150, 100, or 75/minute. Particularly in the case of a rapid, regular supraventricular tachycardia at exactly 150/minute, flutter should be strongly considered even if F waves are not observed.

Although the rate of the F waves — 220 to 300/minute — tends to overlap very little with the usual rate of PAT — 160 to 220/minute — the electrocardiographic distinction is made not on the basis of rate but on the basis of lack of isoelectric baseline and continuously undulating F waves in flutter, as compared with the discrete P waves of PAT. F waves can be small and difficult to find; leads aVF and V_1 are generally the best leads to examine.

Carotid sinus massage to increase the degree of AV block and slow the QRS rate is sometimes invaluable in making F waves obvious for diagnosis. F waves must be absolutely identical in all portions of the tracing before one can make the diagnosis of flutter. At times, coarse atrial fibrillation may somewhat resemble flutter, and a rhythm with ECG characteristics of both may be termed "flutter-fibrillation" (Atlas ECG 5-10); clinically, this rhythm behaves like atrial fibrillation.

Atrial fibrillation results from random chaotic depolarization of the atria. There is no organized electrical activity and, as a consequence, no effective pumping action of the atria. On the ECG, the baseline may be either coarsely or finely irregular (Plate 11J, Atlas ECG 5-11). In some cases, the atrial depolarizations are so small that no activity can be discerned and the baseline appears isoelectric; in such cases, atrial fibrillation is inferred from the irregularly irregular nature of the QRS complexes.

The classic precursor of both atrial flutter and atrial fibrillation is rheumatic disease, especially of the mitral valve, although atherosclerotic disease is a common cause. Atrial fibrillation also may occur in hyperthyroidism, pericarditis, and a host of other diseases, as well as in the sick sinus syndrome in the elderly.

If QRS complexes are regular and narrow, denoting a supraventricular rhythm, and P waves are impossible to discern, a *junctional*, or *nodal*, *rhythm* is likely. Cells of the AV node or, more precisely, at the junction of the atrium and the AV node, are capable of depolarizing spontaneously and becoming the site of origin of the cardiac rhythm. The intrinsic rate of junctional cells is normally 40 to 55/minute — lower than that of the SA node. Thus, the heart is usually controlled by the SA node. However, particularly in cases of SA node dysfunction, the AV node may take over with a junctional rhythm.

Impulses that originate in the AV node are transmitted in a retrograde direction to the atrium and produce P waves, which may well be inverted in leads II, III and aVF. The same impulses are transmitted in an antegrade (forward) direction to the ventricles through the ventricular conduction system. In some cases, the junctional impulse reaches and depolarizes the atrium before the ventricles, in which case the P wave precedes the QRS, although often by a shorter interval or with a different P wave axis than would be expected in sinus rhythm.

If the junctional impulse reaches the atrium and the ventricle at the same time, the P wave of atrial depolarization occurs at the same time as the QRS complex of ventricular depolarization. Since the QRS complex is so much larger, the P wave is buried and often lost in the QRS complex, so that it appears that no P waves are present (Atlas ECG 5-12). If the junctional impulse reaches the ventricles slightly before its retrograde transmission to the atria, the QRS may actually precede the P wave, as in the example in Plate 11K (Atlas ECG 5-13).

Junctional rhythms are sometimes more rapid than the intrinsic junctional rate of 40 to 55/minute and then may be termed *junctional tachycardia* (Atlas ECG 5-14). (Some authorities use the term "tachycardia" only when the rate exceeds 100.) Junctional rhythm or tachycardia, usually at a rate of 80 to 120/minute, is often associated with the acute stage of myocardial infarction but rarely causes hemodynamic problems and is generally not considered dangerous. Junctional rhythm or tachycardia is also a common manifestation of digitalis toxicity. However, when junctional rhythm occurs at the intrinsic junctional tissue rate of 40 to 55/minute in the absence of digitalis or other drugs that may affect cardiac rate or conduction, it is usually an escape rhythm due to poor function of the SA node and can be lifesaving (page 38).

Ventricular Rhythms

The major differential consideration concerning ventricular depolarization is whether the ventricle was activated from a sinoatrial, atrial, or atrioventricular source (all termed "supraventricular") or whether the ventricle was activated from automatic cells within the ventricle (including the Purkinje system) itself. This is of considerable importance, since supraventricular rhythms tend to be much more stable than ventricular rhythms. Furthermore, the intrinsic rate of pacemaker sites tends to decrease, moving from the SA node to the AV node to the ventricle — the order in which alternate pacemakers take over. Diagnosis of a ventricular origin of a rhythm implies either malfunction of all other potential rhythms that should have taken over before a ventricular rhythm or a dangerous irritability of the ventricle, which allows it to take over, usually at a faster rate, even though other sites are still functional.

The differential between supraventricular and ventricular rhythm is made on the basis of the duration (width) of the QRS complex. A narrow QRS complex, one with a duration of less than 0.10 second (less than two and one-half small boxes), means that the entire ventricular myocardium was depolarized quickly. This can occur only if electrical activation spreads along the ventricular conduction system, which is specialized for rapid conduction of activation. The conduction system can be entered only at its origin, that is, at the bundle of His, and so any impulse traversing the conduction system must originate from a supraventricular focus — the SA node, the atrium, or the AV node (junction) (Plate 12A).

A wide QRS (duration more than 0.10 second) indicates that electrical activation required considerable time to spread throughout the ventricular myocardium and thus presumably did not use the ventricular conduction system. There are several possible explanations for this occurrence.

One cause of a wide QRS complex is a defect in intraventricular conduction. A lesion in the ventricular conduction system will result in a slower spread of activation throughout the ventricles and thus a wide QRS. Examples of intraventricular conduction defects are bundle branch blocks, either right or left. The fact that an intraventricular conduction defect is the cause of a wide QRS, even though the impulses originated from a supraventricular site, is usually clear from normal P waves and PR intervals preceding each abnormal QRS (Plate 12B,1; see also Atlas ECGs 6-3 and 6-5).

One unusual cause of a wide QRS complex is the *Wolff-Parkinson-White (WPW) (preexcitation) syndrome* (Plate 12B,2; Atlas ECGs 5-15 and 5-16). Again, the supraventricular origin of the rhythm is generally recognized because of the presence of normal, regular P waves. One is often alerted to the presence of an unusual electrical condition when the PR interval is found to be abnormally short, less than 0.12 second. Measurement of QRS shows it to be abnormally long — more than 0.12 second — but, in addition, a slurred upstroke known as a delta wave is often seen in one or more leads.

The WPW syndrome is due to an abnormal route of conduction from atria to ventricles that bypasses the AV node. In many cases, a particular group of muscle fibers called the bundle of Kent is responsible, but there are many possible abnormal bypass tracts. In the WPW syndrome, impulses generally originate in the SA node, depolarize the atria, produce P waves, and then pass very quickly through the bypass tract without the delay that supraventricular impulses normally experience at the AV node. A small portion of ventricular myocardium is thus excited early ("preexcitation"), producing the early slurred upstroke (the delta wave) of the QRS complex. After the normal delay at the AV node, the sinoatrial impulse also arrives at

Plate 12

Ventricular Rhythms

A. QRS <0.10 second
Supraventricular rhythm with normal intraventricular conduction

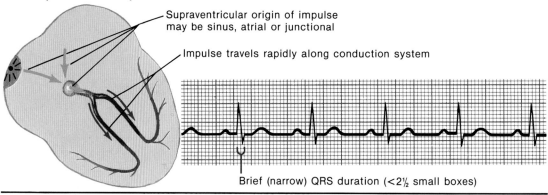

Supraventricular origin of impulse
may be sinus, atrial or junctional

Impulse travels rapidly along conduction system

Brief (narrow) QRS duration (<2½ small boxes)

B. QRS >0.10 second
1. Intraventricular conduction defect (IVCD), including right or left bundle branch block

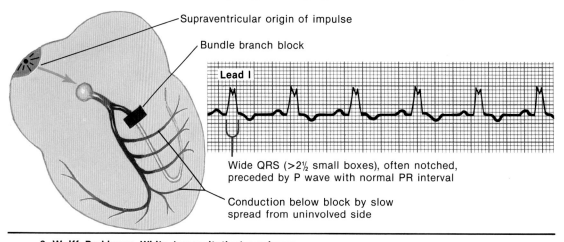

Supraventricular origin of impulse

Bundle branch block

Lead I

Wide QRS (>2½ small boxes), often notched,
preceded by P wave with normal PR interval

Conduction below block by slow
spread from uninvolved side

2. Wolff-Parkinson-White (preexcitation) syndrome

Impulses originate at SA node
and preexcite peripheral
conduction system and ventricular
muscle via bundle of Kent
without delay at AV node.
(In type B, impulses may pass
via posterior accessory bundle)

After normal delay at AV node,
impulses also arrive at
ventricles via normal route to
continue depolarization

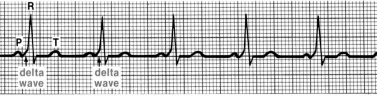

R

P   T

delta wave   delta wave

P wave is immediately followed
by short delta wave, producing
slurred upstroke on wide QRS
with short or no PR interval

Plate 13

Ventricular Rhythms (continued)

B. QRS >0.10 second (continued)

    3. No P waves (ventricular impulse origin)

        a. Rate <40/minute: idioventricular rhythm

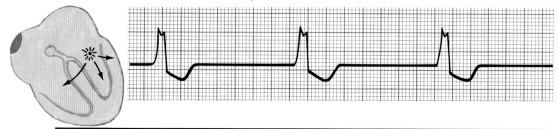

        b. Rate 40 to 120: accelerated idioventricular rhythm (AIVR)

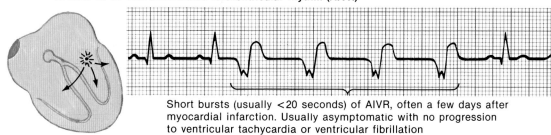

Short bursts (usually <20 seconds) of AIVR, often a few days after myocardial infarction. Usually asymptomatic with no progression to ventricular tachycardia or ventricular fibrillation

        c. Rate >120: ventricular tachycardia

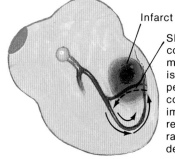

Infarct

Slowed conduction in margin of ischemic area permits circular course of impulse and reentry with rapid repetitive depolarization

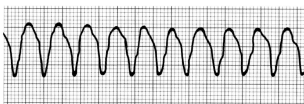

Rapid, bizarre, wide QRS complexes

d. Ventricular fibrillation

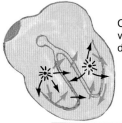

Chaotic ventricular depolarization

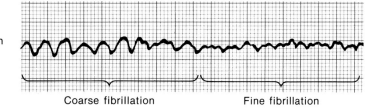

Coarse fibrillation   Fine fibrillation

e. Pacer rhythm

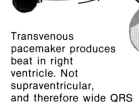

Transvenous pacemaker produces beat in right ventricle. Not supraventricular, and therefore wide QRS

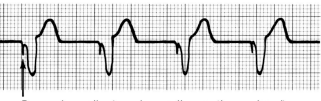

Pacemaker spike (may be small; sometimes missed)

the ventricles via the normal conduction system. Thus, the QRS tends to be prolonged, not because it lasted longer, but because it started earlier as a result of preexcitation. The WPW syndrome is an uncommon cause of a wide (prolonged) QRS that is recognizable because of the associated short PR interval and the unusual slurred onset of the QRS that is known as the delta wave.

If the QRS is longer than 0.10 second and neither an intraventricular conduction defect nor the WPW syndrome seems a likely cause, the rhythm may originate from the ventricle itself. If QRS complexes are wide, often somewhat bizarre, generally with T waves opposite in direction to that of the QRS complex, and with a rate of 20 to 40/minute, *idioventricular rhythm* is diagnosed (Plate 13B,3a; Atlas ECG 5-17). Wide, often bizarre QRS complexes at 40 to 140/minute, most commonly at rates between 80 and 120/minute, constitute *accelerated idioventricular rhythm (AIVR)*, or "slow ventricular tachycardia" (Plate 13B,3b; Atlas ECG 5-18). This disorder often develops in the first few days after acute myocardial infarction. It often occurs in short bursts and usually lasts less than 20 seconds. The patient commonly experiences no symptoms; however, the arrhythmia is often alarming to nurses and physicians because of its resemblance to ventricular tachycardia. There is considerable controversy as to whether AIVR is totally benign; it is clearly less dangerous than ventricular tachycardia, and many authorities do not institute aggressive antiarrhythmic therapy.

Rapid, broad, and often bizarre QRS complexes, with T waves usually opposite in direction to the main QRS deflection and with the rates above 140/minute, are diagnosed as *ventricular tachycardia*. It is thought that many cases of ventricular tachycardia are due to reentry with unidirectional block and slowing of impulse conduction caused by an ischemic area of myocardium (Plate 13B,3c; Atlas ECGs 5-19 and 5-20, first portion).

Chaotic depolarization in the ventricle causes loss of organized QRS complexes (and also loss of organized ventricular contractions); circulatory arrest occurs within seconds. This condition is *ventricular fibrillation*, the cause of most sudden cardiac deaths. Fibrillation may be associated with either coarse or fine chaotic undulations of the ECG baseline, but no true QRS complexes are seen (Plate 13B,3d; Atlas ECG 5-20, latter portion). Ventricular fibrillation is associated with almost immediate loss of consciousness and death within minutes; if a patient is awake, responsive, not in shock, and QRS complexes are not seen, this must be artifactual and is due to problems with electrode attachment, the monitor or cables, or the ECG machine.

The other rhythm that invariably causes almost immediate circulatory arrest and death within a few minutes is *ventricular standstill* (Atlas ECG 5-21). Lethal as it is if untreated, ventricular fibrillation can sometimes be a random electrical phenomenon in an otherwise functional heart, and many patients with ventricular fibrillation have survived immediate electrical defibrillation or cardiopulmonary resuscitation (CPR) with early defibrillation. Ventricular standstill, by contrast, is usually associated with such massive myocardial damage that no rhythm can be generated or sustained anywhere in the ventricles. In many cases, ventricular standstill appears to be the end stage of many minutes of untreated cardiac arrest that began as ventricular fibrillation, and even the disorganized fibrillatory activity disappears as the heart's metabolic and physiologic status becomes terminal.

Ventricular parasystole is an unusual and uncommon arrhythmia resulting from the periodic depolarization of a focus within the ventricles that is "protected" from depolarization by the sinus node or other source of the primary cardiac rhythm. Since the sinus or other primary rhythm is usually faster, most QRS complexes are related to the primary rhythm, and the parasystolic focus is able to "capture" the heart only when it fires between complexes of the primary rhythm, far enough away from complexes of the primary rhythm so that the ventricles are not refractory. The parasystolic complexes are thus intermittent, often occurring at irregular and infrequent intervals on the tracing. Even though the parasystolic focus itself is depolarizing regularly, it simply cannot manage to capture the ventricle more than occasionally.

One other cause of wide QRS complexes is a *ventricular pacemaker rhythm* (Plate 13B,3e). If the pacing wire is located in the ventricle, the origin of the cardiac rhythm is obviously ventricular and the QRS duration will be long. The pacemaker discharge itself produces a pacemaker "spike," which is seen on the ECG as a narrow vertical line at the onset of the broad QRS complex. Pacemaker spikes may be quite small, and if the ECG stylus is not recording heavy lines or if the reader is careless, the pacemaker spike may be missed and a ventricular rhythm erroneously diagnosed. (For a more complete discussion of the electrocardiographic manifestations of artificial cardiac pacemakers, see pages 78–87.)

Atrioventricular Conduction

Atrioventricular conduction is assessed by examining the relationship between the P waves and the QRS complexes (Plate 14). The basic question to be asked is whether P waves are *always* related to QRS complexes, *sometimes* related to QRS complexes, or *never* related to QRS complexes.

If P waves always precede QRS complexes by a fixed *normal* PR interval (0.12 to 0.20 second), AV conduction is normal and *normal sinus rhythm* is the diagnosis.

If P waves always precede QRS complexes but the PR interval is *short* (<0.12 second), there are two possibilities. One is that the supraventricular site of origin is closer than usual to the ventricles — this generally means a *junctional* or *coronary sinus (nonsinus atrial) rhythm*. The other possibility is that atrial activation is being transmitted with unusual rapidity to the ventricle, through the bypass tract, in the preexcitation or the *WPW syndrome*.

If P waves always precede QRS complexes but PR intervals are *variable*, then supraventricular activation is presumed to originate from varying sites, characteristic of *wandering atrial pacemaker* or *multifocal atrial tachycardia*.

If P waves always precede QRS complexes, but the PR interval is *prolonged* (longer than 0.20 second), the diagnosis is *first-degree AV block* (Plate 14D, Atlas ECG 5-22). This is generally a minor AV conduction defect, in which atrial activation is *always* transmitted to the ventricles, although with the unusual delay at or below the AV node.

Progressive lengthening of the PR interval with intermittent dropped beats is characteristic of *second-degree AV block of the Mobitz type I (Wenckebach)* variety (Plate 14E, Atlas ECG 5-23). Second-degree AV block

Plate 14

Atrioventricular Conduction Variations

A. Fixed normal PR interval
   Sinus rhythm (see Plate 10 A)

B. Fixed but short PR interval
   1. **Junctional or coronary sinus rhythm** (see Plate 11 K)
   2. **Wolff-Parkinson-White syndrome** (see Plate 12 B,2)

C. P wave related to each QRS complex, but variable PR interval
   1. **Wandering atrial pacemaker** (see Plate 10 F)
   2. **Multifocal atrial tachycardia** (see Plate 11 G)

D. Fixed but prolonged PR interval
   First-degree AV block

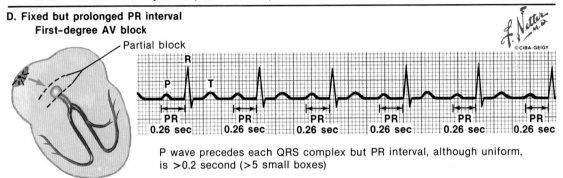

P wave precedes each QRS complex but PR interval, although uniform,
is >0.2 second (>5 small boxes)

E. Progressive lengthening of PR interval with intermittent dropped beats
   Second-degree AV block: Mobitz I (Wenckebach)

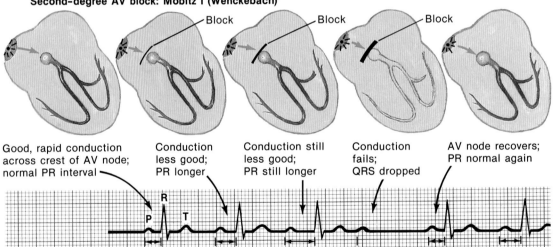

Good, rapid conduction across crest of AV node; normal PR interval

Conduction less good; PR longer

Conduction still less good; PR still longer

Conduction fails; QRS dropped

AV node recovers; PR normal again

F. Sudden dropped QRS without prior PR lengthening
   Second-degree AV block: Mobitz II (non-Wenckebach)

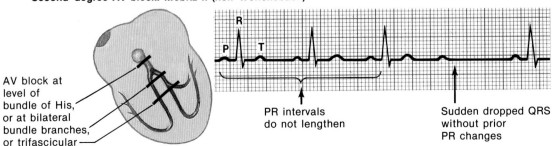

AV block at level of bundle of His, or at bilateral bundle branches, or trifascicular

PR intervals do not lengthen

Sudden dropped QRS without prior PR changes

Plate 15

Atrioventricular Conduction Variations (continued)

G. No relationship between P waves and QRS complexes: QRS rate *slower* than P rate
  Third-degree (complete) AV block

1. Impulses originate at both SA node (P waves) and below site of block in AV node (junctional rhythm) conducting to ventricles

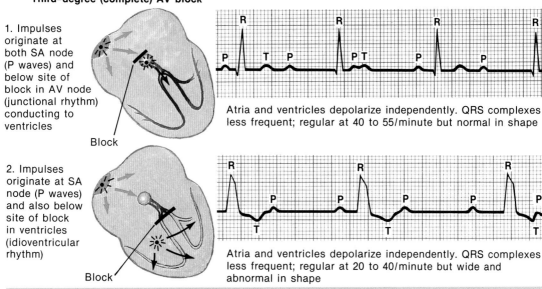

Block

Atria and ventricles depolarize independently. QRS complexes less frequent; regular at 40 to 55/minute but normal in shape

2. Impulses originate at SA node (P waves) and also below site of block in ventricles (idioventricular rhythm)

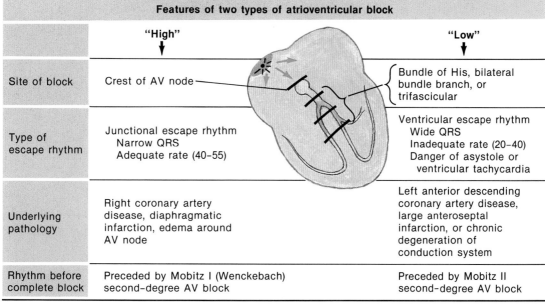

Block

Atria and ventricles depolarize independently. QRS complexes less frequent; regular at 20 to 40/minute but wide and abnormal in shape

Features of two types of atrioventricular block

	"High"	"Low"
Site of block	Crest of AV node	Bundle of His, bilateral bundle branch, or trifascicular
Type of escape rhythm	Junctional escape rhythm Narrow QRS Adequate rate (40-55)	Ventricular escape rhythm Wide QRS Inadequate rate (20-40) Danger of asystole or ventricular tachycardia
Underlying pathology	Right coronary artery disease, diaphragmatic infarction, edema around AV node	Left anterior descending coronary artery disease, large anteroseptal infarction, or chronic degeneration of conduction system
Rhythm before complete block	Preceded by Mobitz I (Wenckebach) second-degree AV block	Preceded by Mobitz II second-degree AV block

H. No relationship between P waves and QRS complexes. QRS rate faster than P rate
  AV dissociation

Slower supraventricular rhythm

Rapid ventricular rhythm, which does not conduct retrograde to atria or shut off sinus

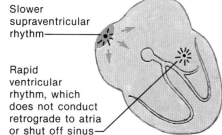

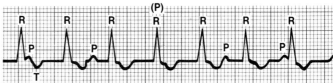

P waves less frequent than QRS complexes and totally unrelated to them

denotes that P waves are *sometimes* related to QRS complexes. Wenckebach was an early-twentieth-century European physician who described the type of second-degree (incomplete) AV block in which the PR interval lengthens progressively and a beat is eventually dropped. Mobitz, a prominent German electrocardiographer, also of the early twentieth century, classified second-degree AV block into the Wenckebach variety with progressive lengthening of the PR interval (now known as Mobitz type I second-degree AV block) and the other variety, Mobitz type II, in which the PR interval is constant and a beat is dropped without warning.

Plate 14E depicts a typical example of Mobitz I (Wenckebach) block. The PR interval is often normal in the first beat of the series, but lengthens progressively with each successive beat until conduction at the AV node fails; a P wave occurs and fails to conduct, and so the QRS is dropped. With a pause between QRS complexes, AV nodal conduction recovers and the next PR interval is short again. This type of second-degree AV block is often further characterized by the number of P waves associated with each set of QRS complexes. In the example shown in Plate 14E, four P waves occur with three QRS complexes; this is called 4:3 Wenckebach. At times, every second beat may be dropped, but more commonly, every third, fourth, fifth, sixth, or only an occasional QRS is dropped.

Recognition of the Mobitz I (Wenckebach) second-degree AV block is extremely important because correlative studies have shown that the site of the anatomic problem is likely to be the crest of the AV node or the junction between the atrium and the AV node itself. This is in contradistinction to Mobitz II (non-Wenckebach) AV block, in which the block is lower.

In Mobitz II AV block, PR intervals are constant, and then a P wave suddenly fails to conduct (Plate 14F, Atlas ECG 5-24). This is another situation in which P waves are *sometimes* related to QRS complexes and thus another example of second-degree or incomplete AV block. Anatomically, Mobitz II AV block tends to occur at the level of the bundle of His, at both bundle branches, or at the level of the three fascicles. (The left bundle has two major divisions, the left anterior and left posterior fascicle; collectively, these two divisions and the right bundle are called the three fascicles.)

When every other QRS complex is dropped, there are never two consecutive PR intervals, and so one cannot determine whether or not the PR interval increases progressively before the dropped beat (Atlas ECG 5-25). This type of second-degree AV block cannot be classified as either Mobitz I or II, and the site of block remains uncertain.

A particularly dangerous type of second-degree heart block is when there are several dropped beats for every conducted beat (Atlas ECG 5-26). This is often termed "high-grade" incomplete heart block. The anatomic lesion is almost invariably below the AV node (as in Mobitz II AV block), and this conduction disturbance is commonly a precursor of complete heart block.

In third-degree, or complete, AV block (Plate 15G,1 and 2), P waves are *never* related to QRS complexes. Although at times a P wave seems to precede a QRS complex by a reasonable interval and one might assume they are related, careful measurement shows that there are two independent rhythms. P waves, at their own regular rate, "march through" the QRS complexes, which are also regular but at a slower rate than the P waves.

The fact that some P waves seem related to QRS complexes is pure coincidence. Complete AV block may occur either just above or below the AV node. If it occurs above or, more precisely, at the crest of the AV node, a junctional rhythm takes over and drives the ventricles, producing narrow QRS complexes at the intrinsic rate of the AV node, usually about 40 to 55/minute (Plate 15G,1; Atlas ECG 5-27). If the site of the complete heart block is below the AV node, the ventricles must be driven from an intrinsic ventricular pacemaker; in this case, the QRS complexes are wide and the rate is the intrinsic rate of a ventricular pacemaker, about 20 to 40/minute (Atlas ECG 5-28).

The tabular material in Plate 15 contrasts two types of AV block — one occurring at the crest of the AV node and the other lower in the conduction system, that is, at the level of the bundle of His, the bundle branches, or the fascicles. Block at the crest of the AV node tends to be much more benign, and is usually preceded by Mobitz I incomplete AV block. In contrast, block lower in the conduction system results either from major damage to the ventricular myocardium from ischemic heart disease — usually extensive anteroseptal infarction — or from chronic degenerative disease of the conduction system. Block lower in the conduction system can be quite dangerous. In the setting of acute myocardial infarction, death often occurs from pump failure (cardiogenic shock) or asystole, even if a pacemaker is inserted.

Complete AV block (or, for that matter, Mobitz II incomplete AV block) associated with acute myocardial infarction is a sign that very large amounts of myocardium have been damaged. In the setting of chronic degenerative disease of the conduction system, *Lenegre's disease*, the prognosis of complete AV block is better, but a permanent pacemaker is often required immediately because the ventricular escape rhythm that occurs in this setting tends to have an inadequate rate and there is some danger of asystole or ventricular tachycardia.

An unusual situation is one in which P waves and QRS complexes occur independently, but the QRS rate is more rapid than the P wave rate. This is called *AV dissociation* (Plate 15H). Failure of a rapid ventricular rhythm to conduct retrograde and to supersede a slower atrial rhythm does not necessarily imply a pathologic condition of the conduction system (as opposed to AV block, in which failure of a more rapid atrial rhythm to conduct antegrade and supersede a slower ventricular rhythm is distinctly abnormal, at least at reasonable heart rates). AV dissociation with more rapid ventricular rates is generally due to unusual irritability of the ventricle itself.

Unusual Complexes

Complexes may be unusual in terms of either timing or contour. If the shape of a QRS complex differs from that of others in the same lead, questions 1, 2, and 3 on pages 20 and 21 can be applied to determine whether the unusual complex is of atrial, junctional, or ventricular origin.

As for timing, unusual complexes may occur early, before the next beat in a regular rhythm is expected, or they may be delayed. Early complexes are called premature contractions. An *atrial premature contraction (APC)* has a narrow QRS (less than 0.10-second duration) and a QRS contour that is generally similar to the normal complexes in all leads. The contour of the P wave of an APC often is slightly different from that of sinus beats, since the origin of the premature contraction and its conduction through the atria are not precisely the same as those of complexes originating from the SA node (Plate 16A,1; Atlas ECG 5-29). The PR interval may be slightly prolonged, presumably because conduction is not occurring through the specialized atrial conduction tracts, but PR intervals of an APC may be normal or even short.

A *junctional premature contraction* (JPC) is also of supraventricular origin. Again, the QRS is narrow, with a contour similar to that of other QRS complexes in all leads. Just as with junctional rhythms, the P wave of a JPC may precede (usually with a short PR interval), be buried in, or follow the QRS (Plate 16A,2; Atlas ECG 5-30).

A *ventricular premature contraction* (VPC) lacks a P wave, and the QRS is wide (more than 0.10 second). The QRS contour is quite different from that of sinus beats in any given lead. A premature contraction with a wide QRS might also be of supraventricular origin with aberrant intraventricular conduction (see Plate 12B and the discussion of intraventricular conduction defects on pages 45–50). At times, the differentiation between a VPC and a supraventricular premature contraction with aberrant intraventricular conduction may be impossible. However, a preceding P wave with a reasonable PR interval favors a supraventricular origin. A contour of the initial portion of the premature contraction similar to that of normal sinus beats in all leads also favors a supraventricular origin with aberrancy. Finally, a premature contraction with a right bundle branch block pattern favors aberrancy, whereas one with a left bundle branch block pattern is more likely to be a VPC (Plate 16A,3; Atlas ECG 5-29, precordial leads).

Premature contractions are probably manifestations of unusual irritability of automatic cells in the atrium, the junctional tissue, or the ventricle, although reentry mechanisms may also be important. In contrast, escape beats occur as a safety mechanism when the sinus or other dominant rhythm temporarily pauses.

The SA node itself may pause, and the rhythm may resume with another sinus beat. If the interval between sinus beats is short (1 to 2 seconds or less), the event is termed a *sinus pause*, while a longer pause is called a *sinus arrest* (Plate 16B). Since the intrinsic rate of automatic firing of the AV node is approximately 40 to 55/minute, corresponding to an interval of 1.2 to 1.6 seconds between complexes, a normal AV node should fire within this period of time if no other site such as the SA node has initiated depolarization. Such activation of the AV node (or junction), caused not by an inherent problem in the AV node but rather by a failure of the SA node or other more rapid pacemaker sites, is a nodal (or junctional) escape beat (Plate 16B, second panel; Atlas ECG 5-31).

Should the SA node *and* the AV node fail, automatic cells in the ventricle must take over or "escape" from their usual control by higher pacemaker sites in order to maintain the heartbeat. The intrinsic rate of automatic cells of the ventricle is 20 to 40/minute, corresponding to an escape interval of 1.8 to 2.2 seconds. Wide, slow QRS complexes with a contour quite different from that of normal sinus beats in all leads are generally ventricular escape beats (Plate 16B, bottom panel; Atlas ECG 5-32).

When dealing with pauses, the electrocardiographer must consider several possible causes. In addition to sinus pause or arrest, a very common reason for a pause is a *blocked APC*, in which the atrial depolarization occurs so soon after the preceding ventricular depolarization that the ventricle is refractory.

Plate 16

Unusual Beats

A. Premature contractions (occur early, before next sinus beat is expected)

1. Atrial

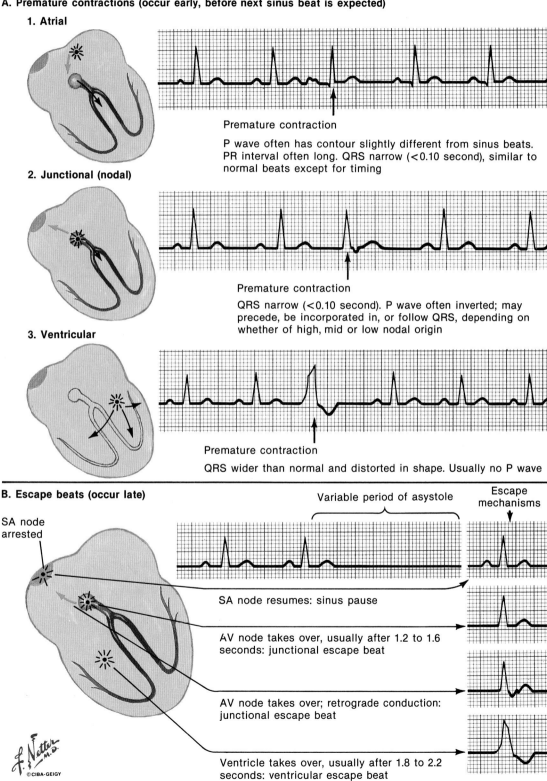

Premature contraction

P wave often has contour slightly different from sinus beats. PR interval often long. QRS narrow (<0.10 second), similar to normal beats except for timing

2. Junctional (nodal)

Premature contraction

QRS narrow (<0.10 second). P wave often inverted; may precede, be incorporated in, or follow QRS, depending on whether of high, mid or low nodal origin

3. Ventricular

Premature contraction

QRS wider than normal and distorted in shape. Usually no P wave

B. Escape beats (occur late)

Variable period of asystole

Escape mechanisms

SA node arrested

SA node resumes: sinus pause

AV node takes over, usually after 1.2 to 1.6 seconds: junctional escape beat

AV node takes over; retrograde conduction: junctional escape beat

Ventricle takes over, usually after 1.8 to 2.2 seconds: ventricular escape beat

Thus, only an extra P wave, without an extra QRS, results (Atlas ECG 5-33). Although the premature atrial depolarization cannot depolarize the refractory ventricle, it does spread backward to depolarize the sinus node, and the sinus must then begin its sequence of depolarization all over again. This results in what is called a "compensatory" pause.

Another unusual situation causing pauses is when the sinus continues to depolarize, but its depolarization is unable to exit from the sinus node for one or more beats and cannot depolarize the atrium, and thus neither P waves nor QRS complexes occur. This rare situation is called *sinus exit block*, and is recognized by pauses that are exact multiples (double, triple, and so forth) of the basic PP interval (Atlas ECG 5-34).

Assessment of Cardiac Arrhythmias

Cardiac arrhythmias are dangerous for several reasons: (1) The rhythm is too slow or potentially too slow, (2) the rhythm is too fast or potentially too fast, or (3) there is serious ventricular irritability.

It is difficult to give hard and fast rules concerning which rate is so slow as to be dangerous. In young athletes, a heart rate in the 40s is not only safe but a sign of excellent physical conditioning, since it indicates a large stroke volume and a consequently slow heart rate. On the other hand, the elderly or those with extensive myocardial disease often cannot increase stroke volume, and cardiac output may fall, sometimes substantially, as a result of an overly slow heart rate. In general, a heart rate below 50/minute, except in young people or athletes, is cause for concern. Such slow ventricular rates might occur with severe sinus bradycardia, slow junctional rhythms, and complete heart block with ventricular escape rhythm.

Rhythms that are dangerous because of their potential for severe bradycardia are those that are often precursors of high-grade AV block. Mobitz I (Wenckebach) second-degree heart block may progress to complete heart block, but generally with a junctional escape rhythm at a rate most often between 40 and 55/minute. Thus, Mobitz I incomplete AV block is not as potentially dangerous as Mobitz II second-degree heart block, in which progression to complete heart block generally results in a ventricular escape rhythm with a very slow heart rate.

The danger from rapid heart rates (tachyarrhythmias) is also variable, depending on age and the extent of cardiac disease. Babies and children routinely have very high heart rates, and young people without cardiac disease can tolerate a heart rate of 150/minute and higher without difficulty. In older patients, who may have clinical or occult atherosclerotic disease, rapid heart rates may be quite dangerous in that they may cause myocardial ischemia. Any tachyarrhythmia is dangerous if it so compromises cardiac output as to produce hypotension or cerebral symptoms such as dizziness or fainting. Any tachyarrhythmia is dangerous when associated with chest pain or other signs of myocardial ischemia such as ST segment depression or ventricular irritability. As a general rule, except in young persons, a heart rate over 150/minute is cause for concern.

Arrhythmias that are dangerous because of their potential for severe tachycardia are those in which the atrial rate is extremely rapid but some degree of AV block maintains a reasonably slow ventricular rate. AV block may decrease and the ventricular rate may increase. In atrial flutter, for example, the atrial rate is usually around 300/minute. Atrial flutter with 3:1 AV block and a ventricular rate of 100/minute is a potentially dangerous arrhythmia if the AV block should decrease to 2:1 or 1:1, in which case the ventricular rate would increase to 150 or even 300/minute. The same concern applies to atrial fibrillation and PAT with some degree of AV block.

The third type of danger concerns ventricular irritability. Sudden cardiac arrest is an all too common cause of death in the United States, occurring over 300,000 times a year. In most cases, sudden cardiac death is caused by ventricular fibrillation, and some ventricular arrhythmias may be harbingers of ventricular fibrillation. Certainly, ventricular tachycardia is in this warning category, and is therefore considered to be highly dangerous. In some circumstances, two or three VPCs in a row (so-called couplets or triplets), multifocal VPCs, so-called R on T VPCs (VPCs that occur so prematurely they fall on the T wave of the preceding QRS complexes), or even large numbers of single VPCs appear to be associated with an increased risk of ventricular fibrillation. Thus, arrhythmias that warn of potential ventricular irritability may also be considered potentially dangerous arrhythmias.

A complete discussion of the danger of ventricular irritability is beyond the scope of this book, but in general, ventricular arrhythmias are most feared when associated with major symptoms (such as hypotension and syncope) or when they occur in the setting of acute ischemic heart disease (myocardial infarction or unstable angina) or decompensated congestive heart failure. Conversely, ventricular arrhythmias may be less ominous, regardless of the electrocardiographic appearance, in patients who do not have structural cardiac disease.

6 CHAMBER ENLARGEMENT AND INTRAVENTRICULAR CONDUCTION DEFECTS

The complete electrocardiographic reading includes not only determination of cardiac rhythm, but also assessment of possible atrial or ventricular enlargement; fascicular or bundle branch blocks; significant Q waves; and other abnormalities of the QRS complex, the ST segment, and T waves.

Right Atrial Enlargement

Examination of pattern abnormalities of the ECG begins with the P wave — its amplitude (height), duration, and contour. In right atrial enlargement (RAE) (sometimes called right atrial hypertrophy [RAH] or right atrial abnormality [RAA]), the P wave is characteristically tall and peaked, particularly in leads II, III and aVF. The usual criterion for right atrial enlargement is P wave amplitude ≥ 2.5 mm. This increased amplitude results from increased electrical forces associated with hypertrophy of right atrial tissue, along with a shift in the direction of the P wave axis downward toward the feet, that is, in the direction of the positive poles of leads II, III and aVF (Plate 17, Atlas ECG 6-1).

Plate 17

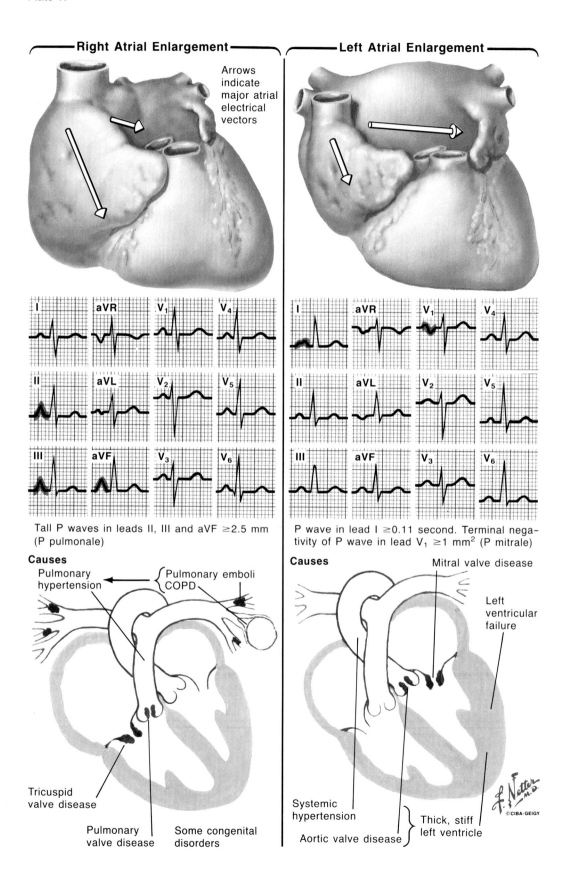

Right Atrial Enlargement

Arrows indicate major atrial electrical vectors

Tall P waves in leads II, III and aVF ≥2.5 mm (P pulmonale)

Causes

Pulmonary hypertension

Pulmonary emboli COPD

Tricuspid valve disease

Pulmonary valve disease

Some congenital disorders

Left Atrial Enlargement

P wave in lead I ≥0.11 second. Terminal negativity of P wave in lead V_1 ≥1 mm^2 (P mitrale)

Causes

Mitral valve disease

Left ventricular failure

Systemic hypertension

Aortic valve disease

Thick, stiff left ventricle

©CIBA-GEIGY

Right atrial enlargement is usually caused by pressure or volume overload of the right atrium, which in turn is associated with tricuspid valvular disease (relatively rare), or by one of the numerous conditions causing pulmonary hypertension. The most common of the latter conditions are severe chronic obstructive pulmonary disease (COPD), pulmonary emboli, and mitral valve stenosis or insufficiency (Plate 17, bottom left).

Since RAE is so frequently caused by pulmonary hypertension, the characteristic tall, peaked P wave associated with RAE is often termed "P pulmonale." In unusual situations in which pulmonary hypertension appears or disappears rapidly (as when a large, acute pulmonary embolus breaks up quickly), P pulmonale also appears and disappears rapidly. Since hypertrophy cannot be an acute phenomenon, it seems better to term the electrocardiographic abnormality "right atrial enlargement" or "right atrial abnormality."

Left Atrial Enlargement

Left atrial enlargement (LAE) is associated with several possible electrocardiographic findings: (1) a wide P wave, ≥ 0.11 second in duration in any ECG lead; (2) a notch or "double hump" in the P wave in any lead, with the two peaks ≥ 0.04 second apart (lead I in Plate 17, middle right); and (3) negative deflection in the terminal portion of the P wave in lead V_1 ≥ 1 mm (0.10 mv) deep and ≥ 1 mm wide (≥ 0.04-second duration) (lead V_1 in Plate 17, middle right; Atlas ECG 6-2). Of these three criteria, the last is the most specific. "Possible LAE" is usually diagnosed if the P wave is either broad or notched, whereas "definite LAE" is diagnosed only when the characteristic terminal negative forces are ≥ 1 mm^2 (1 mm deep $\times$ 1 mm wide) in lead V_1.

In LAE, or left atrial hypertrophy (LAH), the P wave vector is shifted to the left, away from leads II, III, aVF and V_1, where P wave amplitude is normally greatest. Thus, P wave amplitude is not generally increased in LAE. Since atrial depolarization requires more time in enlargement or hypertrophy, the duration of the P wave is increased. In some instances, however, the duration of atrial depolarization appears to be related to abnormalities of the interatrial conduction system rather than to actual anatomic enlargement or hypertrophy of the atrium; thus, the term "left atrial abnormality" (LAA) is often used (although both LAH and LAE are also used in ECG interpretations).

Since LAE is commonly the result of mitral valve stenosis or insufficiency, the broad, notched P wave of LAE is often termed "P mitrale." LAE results from increased work of the left atrium in filling an abnormal left ventricle, and is frequently associated with left ventricular hypertrophy (LVH). Both LAE and LVH are often caused by systemic hypertension, aortic valvular disease, hypertrophic cardiomyopathy, or other conditions that reduce left ventricular compliance (Plate 17, bottom right).

Right Ventricular Hypertrophy

Right ventricular hypertrophy (RVH) is characterized by a tall R wave in lead V_1, along with other evidence of increased right ventricular electrical forces: right axis deviation, relatively taller R waves in the right precordium,

Plate 18

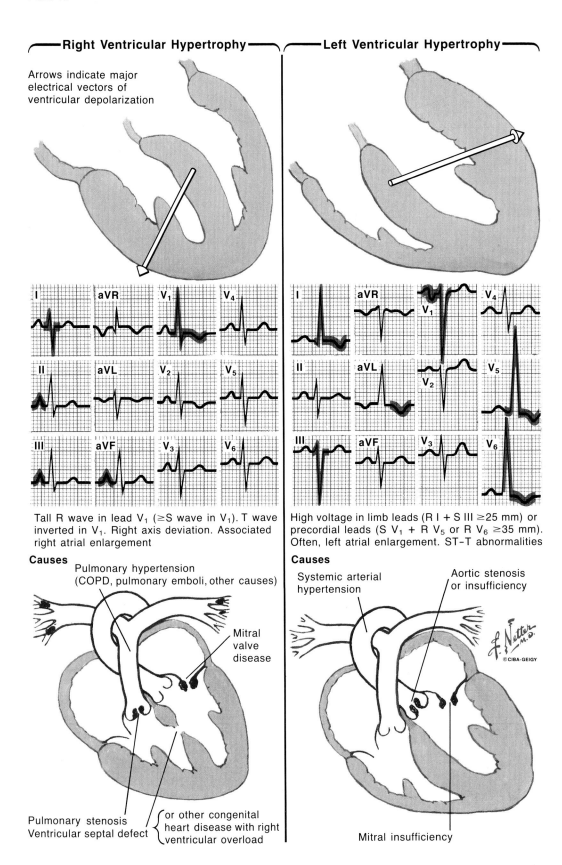

Right Ventricular Hypertrophy

Arrows indicate major electrical vectors of ventricular depolarization

Tall R wave in lead V_1 (≥S wave in V_1). T wave inverted in V_1. Right axis deviation. Associated right atrial enlargement

Causes

Pulmonary hypertension (COPD, pulmonary emboli, other causes)

Mitral valve disease

Pulmonary stenosis
Ventricular septal defect
{or other congenital heart disease with right ventricular overload

Left Ventricular Hypertrophy

High voltage in limb leads (R I + S III ≥25 mm) or precordial leads (S V_1 + R V_5 or R V_6 ≥35 mm). Often, left atrial enlargement. ST–T abnormalities

Causes

Systemic arterial hypertension

Aortic stenosis or insufficiency

Mitral insufficiency

©CIBA-GEIGY

and relatively deeper S waves in the left precordial leads than are normally seen (Plate 18, top left and middle; Atlas ECG 6-1). Initial suspicion of RVH generally arises from examination of the QRS in lead V_1; R wave height exceeding S wave depth in lead V_1 (often abbreviated R≥S V_1) raises the possibility of RVH, as does the finding of an R wave in lead V_1 with absolute amplitude ≥7 mm (0.70 mv). The differential diagnosis of a tall R wave in lead V_1 (R≥S V_1) includes true posterior myocardial infarction and counter-clockwise rotation of the heart. In contrast to these two conditions, RVH is usually associated with right axis deviation, and the T waves in lead V_1 (and sometimes also in leads V_2 and V_3) are inverted.

Deep S waves in left precordial leads such as V_4 through V_6 are common in RVH, representing abnormally large forces of right ventricular depolarization directed away from these left-sided leads. In contradistinction, true posterior myocardial infarction, also manifesting R≥S in lead V_1, is generally accompanied by diaphragmatic myocardial infarction (Q waves or T wave inversions, or both, in leads II, III and aVF); the T wave in lead V_1 is usually upright in true posterior myocardial infarction (page 61, see also Atlas ECG 7-11).

Counterclockwise rotation of the heart (see Atlas ECG 7-12) is a relatively common and usually benign situation in which noncardiac conditions such as abnormalities of the thoracic bones or simply normal biologic variation causes the heart to be rotated in the chest. The interventricular septum is normally positioned under the center of the sternum, so that lead V_1 is to the right of the septum and is located over the right ventricle. Thus, the normal QRS complex in lead V_1 has a smaller R wave (reflecting forces from the closer but smaller right ventricle) and a larger S wave (representing forces of the more distant but larger left ventricle). Lead V_2 is located approximately over the interventricular septum and may reflect either slight right ventricular or slight left ventricular preponderance (either the R wave or the S wave may be taller, and often the two are of approximately equal amplitude).

Leads V_3 through V_6 are normally located over the left ventricle and reflect predominantly left ventricular electrical forces, that is, a relatively large and positive R wave with little if any S wave from the small and distant right ventricle.

Cardiac rotation is conventionally expressed as if one were looking up at the heart from the pelvis. If the heart rotates so that the septum is under lead V_3 or V_4 rather than in its usual position under lead V_2, this is termed "clockwise" rotation; if the septum moves in the other direction so that it is under lead V_1, this is "counterclockwise" rotation. In counterclockwise rotation, if the septum moves toward lead V_1 or beyond, lead V_1 may actually be reflecting mainly left ventricular forces. In this situation, a predominantly positive QRS would be expected, that is, R≥S V_1. This benign situation is differentiated from RVH and posterior myocardial infarction (the other two conditions associated with R≥S V_1) by the absence of any other ECG abnormalities (Table 1).

Right ventricular hypertrophy is caused by abnormalities of the pulmonary valve (which are uncommon in adults) and by conditions that cause pulmonary hypertension (page 41). RVH also can be caused by various congenital lesions that produce either volume or pressure overload of the right ventricle (for example, atrial or ventricular septal defect and many others

Table 1 Differential Diagnosis of Tall R Wave in (R ≥ S V₁)

Diagnosis	Inverted T wave in lead V₁	RAD*	DMI†
Counterclockwise rotation of the heart	±	No	No
True posterior myocardial infarction	No	No	Often
Right ventricular hypertrophy‡	Yes	Yes	No

*RAD = right axis deviation of QRS

†DMI = diaphragmatic myocardial infarction, manifested by Q waves or T wave inversions, or both, in leads II, III, aVF

‡Right atrial enlargement often accompanies RVH and makes the diagnosis of RVH more certain

[Plate 18, bottom left]) and by tricuspid regurgitation, itself often associated with long-standing mitral valve disease. RVH is not associated with tricuspid valve stenosis, which affects only the right atrium.

Left Ventricular Hypertrophy

A number of criteria have been developed for diagnosis of LVH. In general, the most sensitive criteria are not sufficiently specific, and their use may result in overdiagnosis of LVH. Very specific criteria are less sensitive; although they are diagnostic of LVH, many less obvious cases of LVH are missed when such criteria are used. The criteria most commonly used for a diagnosis of LVH were developed many years ago. With the availability of echocardiography, cardiac catheterization, and other accurate ways of assessing ventricular hypertrophy, many new electrocardiographic criteria for LVH have been suggested. Although many laboratories have their own criteria, most are variations of the following four well-accepted standards, which are quite simple to use.

1. Increased QRS voltage in the standard leads, generally measured as the R wave in lead I plus the S wave in lead III ≥25 mm (2.5 mv).
2. Increased precordial voltage: S wave in lead V_1 plus R wave in lead V_5 or V_6 ≥35 mm (3.5 mv).*
3. ST segment and T wave abnormalities (pages 64–78).
4. Left atrial abnormality.

Some authorities add a fifth criterion: R wave amplitude in lead aVL ≥11 mm. Others include R or S wave amplitude in any limb lead ≥20 mm, R wave amplitude in lead V_5 or V_6 ≥30 mm, S wave amplitude in lead V_1 or V_2 ≥30 mm, or marked left axis deviation among the various criteria to be considered in the diagnosis of LVH.

---

*Precordial voltage criteria for LVH apply only to persons over age 40. Higher precordial voltage may be normal in young adults, and voltage is normally very high in children.

A common convention is to diagnose "possible LVH" if any one of the first three criteria is present, "probable LVH" if any two of the four or five criteria are present, and "definite LVH" if any three of the four or five criteria are present (Plate 18, middle right; Atlas ECG 6-2).

Left ventricular hypertrophy is caused by systemic arterial hypertension, stenosis or insufficiency of the aortic valve, mitral valve insufficiency, and various other conditions that lead to volume or pressure overload of the left ventricle (Plate 18, bottom right).

Right Bundle Branch Block

In bundle branch block, ventricular depolarization is abnormal. Normally, impulses from the sinus node, atrium, and AV node proceed through the common bundle of His and then down both left and right bundle branches to the Purkinje fibers, which form the terminal portions of the intraventricular conduction system. If the right bundle branch is blocked, conduction must proceed down the left bundle, and the right ventricle is depolarized by forces coming from the left ventricle, traveling through the myocardial cells of the interventricular septum, and then reaching the right ventricle.

Since the forces traveling across the septum are unable to use the ventricular conduction fibers specialized for rapid conduction of electrical impulses, depolarization of the right ventricle is delayed. This has two consequences. First, more time elapses from the beginning to the end of ventricular depolarization; that is, the QRS complex is prolonged, ≥0.10 second in duration. Second, the electrical forces of right ventricular depolarization are no longer overshadowed and buried within the forces of left ventricular depolarization.

Since the right ventricle is a low-pressure chamber that pumps only to the lungs, the myocardium of the right ventricle is considerably less massive than that of the left, and electrical forces of the right ventricle are normally overshadowed by those from the left ventricle. With right bundle branch block (RBBB) and delay of right ventricular depolarization, the right ventricular forces occur after left ventricular depolarization and become visible as late rightward and anteriorly directed forces (that is, depolarization originating in the left ventricle via the intact left bundle branch and then traveling rightward across the interventricular septum toward the anteriorly situated right ventricle).

Complete RBBB is characterized by prolonged QRS complex (≥0.12 second in duration) and an abnormal late portion of the QRS directed toward the right ventricle and away from the left ventricle (more precisely, terminal rightward and anterior forces ≥0.04 second in duration). This is usually manifested by a broad terminal S wave in lead I and in other leads located over the left precordium such as V_5 and V_6, a terminal broad R wave in lead aVR, and the characteristic so-called RSR' complex (read as "R-S-R-prime") in lead V_1 (Plate 19, top right; Atlas ECG 6-3). The later positive deflection, the R', may be either smaller or larger in amplitude than the initial, often small R wave in lead V_1 that represents the normal early septal depolarization from left to right.

Plate 19

Right Bundle Branch Block

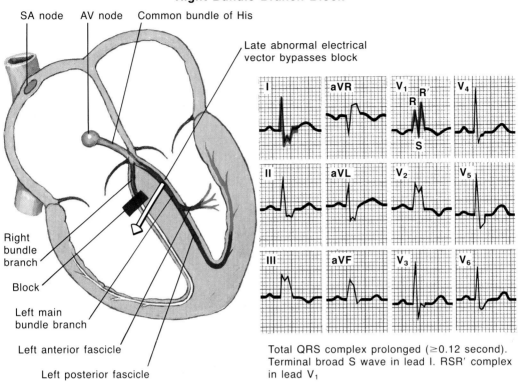

SA node · AV node · Common bundle of His

Late abnormal electrical
vector bypasses block

Right
bundle
branch

Block

Left main
bundle branch

Left anterior fascicle

Left posterior fascicle

Total QRS complex prolonged ($\geq$0.12 second).
Terminal broad S wave in lead I. RSR′ complex
in lead V_1

Left Bundle Branch Block

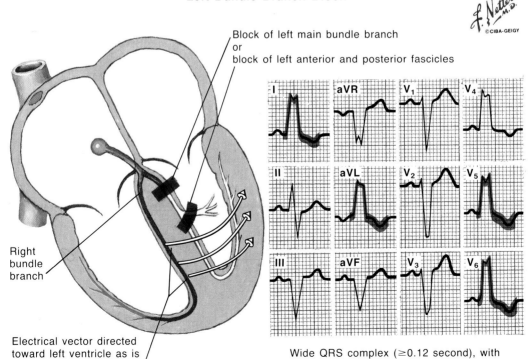

Block of left main bundle branch
or
block of left anterior and posterior fascicles

Right
bundle
branch

Electrical vector directed
toward left ventricle as is
normal, but delayed and
prolonged

Wide QRS complex ($\geq$0.12 second), with
ST depressions and inverted T waves,
particularly in leads I, aVL, V_5 and V_6

If the RBBB is caused by anteroseptal infarction, the initial septal forces disappear, so that the R wave is absent and the complex in lead V_1 may be simply an early Q and a late R wave (in this case, the late R wave directed toward the right ventricle represents the same delayed forces coming across the interventricular septum as the R′ in the RSR′ complex of RBBB). At times, there may be no return to baseline between the R wave and the R′; this produces a broad QRS complex that has two notches and looks something like the letter "M" (lead V_2 in both Plate 19, top right, and Atlas ECG 6-3).

The normal QRS duration is <0.10 second; a QRS duration of 0.10 or 0.11 second is borderline, neither normal nor definitely abnormal. In past years, an RSR′ pattern and QRS duration in the gray area from 0.10 to 0.11 second was designated "incomplete" bundle branch block, but since it is unclear whether there is any anatomic entity of "incomplete" bundle branch block, this term has recently fallen into disfavor. This poses a problem, since no accepted electrocardiographic diagnosis has replaced the old term. In such situations, ECG readers sometimes must use terms such as "borderline" or "incomplete" within quotation marks to indicate that the diagnosis is only a description of the ECG and may not accurately reflect the anatomic abnormality.

Sometimes, the designation "right ventricular conduction defect" is used to describe a QRS pattern that resembles RBBB without a prolonged QRS complex (Atlas ECG 6-4).

The right bundle is a relatively thin bundle of conduction fibers and is more vulnerable to interruption than the left bundle, which branches early and widely. Thus, RBBB may not imply myocardial damage as serious and as widespread as in block of the left bundle branch. RBBB may be caused by relatively small anatomic lesions, although the most usual causes are idiopathic degenerative conduction system disease (causing fibrosis and interruption of the conduction fibers) and ischemic heart disease in the anterior septum where the right bundle courses.

Left Bundle Branch Block

The consequences of complete left bundle branch block (LBBB) are similar but opposite to those of RBBB. Since the left ventricle cannot be normally depolarized from the left bundle, depolarization must proceed down the right bundle and across the interventricular septum from the right to the left ventricle. Again, since this abnormal depolarization proceeds via myocardial rather than specialized conduction fibers, it takes longer, so that the QRS complex is widened and the duration is prolonged (≥0.12 second).

In contradistinction to RBBB, in LBBB the abnormal forces proceeding across the septum are traveling from right to left, which is the same direction as most forces during normal ventricular depolarization. Thus, the QRS complex in LBBB, although bizarre in appearance, has the same general orientation as in normal depolarization. In LBBB, the QRS complex is always wide but has many variations in shape (Plate 19, bottom right; Atlas ECG 6-5). The following are commonly seen: notches in the QRS complex; unusually high voltage; either deep S waves in lead V_1, V_2 or V_3 or tall R waves in lead I, aVL, V_5 or V_6; left axis deviation of the QRS complex, which may be marked; very small R waves in leads V_1 through V_3, sometimes so small that the QRS looks like a QS complex and anterior or anteroseptal myocardial infarction may be erroneously diagnosed; and some delay in the time from onset of the QRS to its peak amplitude, manifested as a less steep upstroke of the initial portion of the QRS. This initial upstroke has been called the "intrinsicoid deflection," and a "delayed intrinsicoid deflection" has been cited as a feature of LBBB; however, this term is now rarely used.

In LBBB, the small septal Q wave that is normally seen in leads I, aVL, V_5 and V_6 disappears. A prominent electrocardiographic feature of LBBB is the pronounced and often bizarre ST segment and T wave abnormalities. These commonly take the form of ST segment depressions and T wave inversions, often marked, in a direction opposite to the main QRS complex in most leads (Plate 19, bottom right; Atlas ECG 6-5).

Since the left bundle branches early and widely throughout the left ventricle, complete LBBB usually indicates widespread myocardial disease. It, too, may occur with degenerative conduction system disease, ischemic heart disease, or a number of conditions that produce major LVH.

In both RBBB and LBBB, the underlying heart disease that produced the block rather than the conduction abnormality itself usually determines prognosis. In a very few persons, bundle branch block develops in the absence of any apparent heart disease. If cardiac catheterization and coronary angiography prove that there is indeed no structural heart disease, morbidity and mortality appear to be extremely low over many years.

Left Anterior Fascicular Block

The left bundle branch divides into two major divisions: the left anterior fascicle and the left posterior fascicle. Block of the left anterior fascicle is relatively common and is usually termed "left anterior hemiblock" (LAH). As with the bundle branch blocks, with left anterior fascicular block, depolarization must reach the portion of the heart normally served by this fascicle from other areas that have been normally depolarized. In the case of the hemiblocks, spread of electrical activity into the blocked areas does not prolong overall depolarization, and so the QRS complex is of normal duration. It also is generally of normal shape, without unusual notching, delayed upstroke, or ST segment or T wave abnormalities (Plate 20, top). In LAH, however, the QRS axis is shifted far to the left, and the diagnosis is made solely from the finding of marked left axis deviation (QRS axis is more negative than $-30°$, which gives a predominantly negative deflection or S wave > R wave in leads II, III and aVF in the absence of diaphragmatic myocardial infarction). (See Plate 9, bottom right, for review of marked left axis deviation, and Atlas ECG 6-3, which shows LAH but also has an abnormal QRS caused by RBBB, not LAH.)

Left anterior hemiblock is most often caused by either degenerative conduction system disease or ischemic heart disease. Unless it occurs in the context of acute myocardial infarction, it is usually benign and is only rarely a precursor of complete LBBB in the short term.

Left Posterior Fascicular Block

As with the other ventricular conduction defects, block of the left posterior fascicle of the left bundle (often termed "left posterior hemiblock" [LPH]) leads to depolarization of tissue in the area beyond the block from other

Plate 20

Left Anterior Fascicular Block

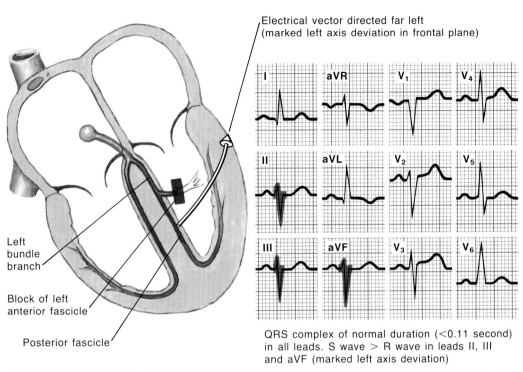

Electrical vector directed far left
(marked left axis deviation in frontal plane)

Left bundle branch

Block of left anterior fascicle

Posterior fascicle

QRS complex of normal duration (<0.11 second) in all leads. S wave > R wave in leads II, III and aVF (marked left axis deviation)

Left Posterior Fascicular Block

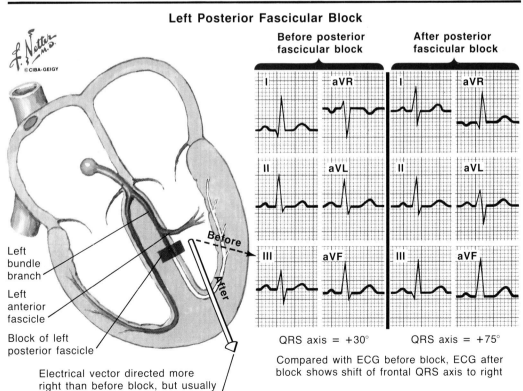

Before posterior fascicular block

After posterior fascicular block

Left bundle branch

Left anterior fascicle

Block of left posterior fascicle

Before

After

Electrical vector directed more right than before block, but usually within normal QRS axis range

QRS axis = +30°

QRS axis = +75°

Compared with ECG before block, ECG after block shows shift of frontal QRS axis to right

normally activated sections of myocardium. In LPH, as in LAH, this abnormal depolarization proceeds quickly and the QRS complex is not prolonged. However, the electrical axis of the QRS shifts toward the right in LPH.

LPH is more difficult to diagnose than LAH, since the rightward shift of the QRS axis is often not very striking, and the final axis often remains within the normal range. Thus, if the QRS duration and axis are normal in LPH, the condition cannot be diagnosed from a single ECG. Two tracings are needed, one before the block and the other showing the QRS axis shift to the right (Plate 20, bottom right).

Some authorities require more stringent criteria for LPH, namely, a QRS axis $\geq +120°$ in the absence of RVH or anterolateral myocardial infarction (Atlas ECG 6-6). In any case, LPH is hardly ever diagnosed on a routine ECG, partly because of difficulty in recognition and partly because it seems to be quite uncommon. Like LAH, LPH is most commonly due to degenerative conduction system disease or ischemic heart disease and seems relatively benign unless it occurs in the context of acute myocardial infarction.

Because the left bundle branch has two major divisions and the right bundle branch provides a third pathway for AV conduction, the concept of three fascicles is now commonly used in describing AV conduction. Thus, there may be abnormalities of conduction in one fascicle (LAH, LPH, or RBBB); in two fascicles (LAH or LPH *plus* RBBB, frequently referred to as "bifascicular block"); or even in all three fascicles (usually LAH plus RBBB *plus* prolonged PR interval >0.20 second or first-degree AV block, which represents disease in the sole remaining avenue for AV conduction [Atlas ECG 6-3]). Note that LBBB (which is LAH plus LPH) is also a type of bifascicular block, and LBBB plus first-degree AV block is a type of trifascicular block, although the terms "bifascicular block" and "trifascicular block" in clinical practice almost always refer to LAH plus RBBB and LAH plus RBBB plus first-degree AV block, respectively.

Bifascicular block and trifascicular block are common electrocardiographic abnormalities and occur frequently in patients in whom more severe AV conduction abnormalities, including second- or third-degree (complete) heart block, eventually develop. However, many more patients display the electrocardiographic abnormality of bifascicular block or trifascicular block for years or even all their life without ever having more severe or dangerous conduction problems. Thus, although bifascicular block and trifascicular block certainly indicate more severe conduction system disease and may prompt closer follow-up or further diagnostic testing, they are *not* generally considered indications for permanent pacemaker insertion in the asymptomatic patient.

Aside from RBBB and LBBB, there are other situations in which the QRS duration is prolonged despite a sinus or other supraventricular pacemaker. These ECGs have a QRS complex with a duration of ≥ 0.10 second but without specific features of either RBBB or LBBB. Such ECGs are diagnosed as intraventricular conduction defect (IVCD), and QRS complexes vary widely from IVCDs of RBBB type to those of LBBB type, with some bearing no resemblance whatever to either of the bundle branch blocks (Atlas ECG 6-7). Note that RBBB, LBBB, LAH, and LPH are all types of IVCD, but the electrocardiographic diagnosis IVCD has come to represent a "wastebasket" designation for all those IVCDs that cannot be characterized more precisely.

Plate 21

Differential Diagnosis of Q Waves

| ── Nonsignificant ── | ── Significant ── |

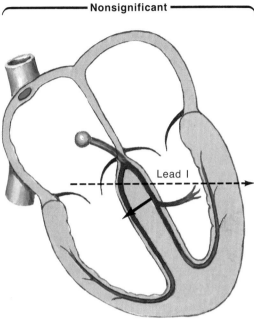

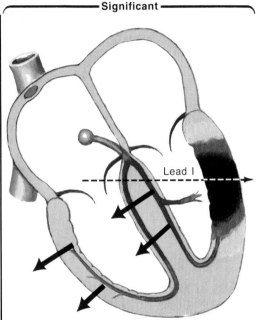

Q wave is normally produced in lead I by initial depolarization of interventricular septum, with electrical vector directed to right and downward. Septum is relatively thin and depolarization occurs quickly, generating only small, short–lived potential

In myocardial infarction, dead muscle tissue produces no action potential, and electrocardiograph "looks through" infarcted area to pick up electrical forces from opposite side of heart, which are directed away from lead I

Resultant septal Q wave in lead I is of small amplitude (<25% of succeeding R wave) and short duration (<0.04 second, ie, <1 small box on ECG tracing)

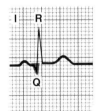

Q wave in myocardial infarction is accordingly of substantial amplitude (≥25% of R wave) and duration (≥0.04 second)

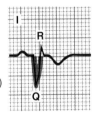

Q wave in idiopathic hypertrophic subaortic stenosis (IHSS)

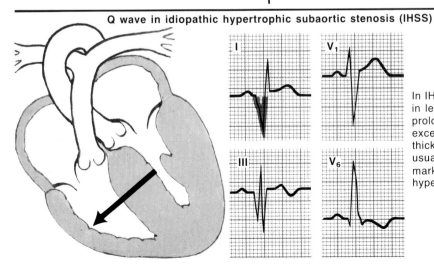

In IHSS, septal Q wave in lead I is deep and prolonged because of excessive septal thickness. Other leads usually evidence marked left ventricular hypertrophy

7 MYOCARDIAL INFARCTION AND ISCHEMIA

Myocardial infarction and ischemia are characterized by abnormalities in three portions of the ECG: Q waves, ST segments, and T waves. After assessment of cardiac rhythm, rate, axis, atrial and ventricular enlargement, bundle branch blocks, and fascicular blocks, a search is generally made for abnormalities of the QRS complex, the ST segment, and the T wave, in that order. The electrocardiographer first generally considers the Q wave, the initial negative deflection of the QRS complex.

Small Q waves are normal, the result of depolarization of the interventricular septum from left to right. This produces electrical forces directed away from the left ventricle, or initial negative forces in leads I, aVL, V_5 and V_6. However, the normal septum is relatively thin, and its depolarization occurs quickly (within 0.04 second) and produces forces of low amplitude. The resultant normal "septal Q wave" is thus less than 0.04 second wide and of low amplitude, often defined as a Q wave depth less than 25% of the height of the succeeding R wave (Plate 21, top left; Atlas ECG 7-1).

The Q wave in myocardial infarction has quite a different origin. Infarcted myocardium produces no electrical potentials and thus little or nothing in the way of electrical forces directed toward an electrode overlying the infarction. In this case, most electrical activity, particularly from the opposite, noninfarcted wall of the heart is traveling away from the electrode positioned over an infarction, and thus such an electrode detects primarily negative electrical forces, producing a large Q wave (Plate 21, top right; see also Atlas ECGs 7-7, 7-9, 7-10, and 7-11).

The size of a normal septum that produces the nonsignificant septal Q wave and the extent of a myocardial infarction that might produce a "significant" Q wave vary somewhat among individuals. In general, the stricter the criteria for significance of a Q wave, the more accurate (specific) are such criteria in the diagnosis of definite myocardial infarction. However, strict criteria are less sensitive, and with use of such criteria, some small infarctions may not be diagnosed. Conversely, looser criteria for "significant" Q waves are more sensitive, and their application results in detection of a larger proportion of infarctions. However, with use of the looser criteria, there is less certainty that every diagnosis of an infarction is accurate.

The novice electrocardiographer is likely to find the following "rules" and "criteria" for "significant" Q waves confusing, complex, and maddening in their imprecision. Unfortunately, there is no single recognized authoritative body that sets standards for ECG interpretation. In addition, new diagnostic methods to validate an electrocardiographic diagnosis are constantly becoming available. The vectorcardiogram (VCG), for example, is probably a bit more accurate in the diagnosis of myocardial infarction than the standard ECG, but it is more expensive and more difficult to perform and interpret. Thus, the VCG is becoming less and less available, even in large hospitals. The echocardiogram, radionuclide techniques such as thallium perfusion scanning and gated blood pool imaging, and cardiac catheterization are also quite useful in the diagnosis of myocardial infarction, but these tests are not perfect either. Thus, various invasive and noninvasive methods used to validate electrocardiographic findings may sometimes have slightly different results.

Despite all the recent advances in diagnostic techniques and electrocardiographic research in the diagnosis of myocardial infarction, most electrocardiographers use some adaptation of a classification system originally developed for epidemiologic studies more than two decades ago by Henry Blackburn and associates at the University of Minnesota, a system familiarly known as the "Minnesota Code." Although the full computer coding system is much too complicated for everyday use, the criteria listed here have been adapted from the code and represent a reasonable approximation of what most electrocardiographers use. The following are general rules concerning Q waves.

1. Q waves are never significant in lead aVR, and this lead is never examined for Q waves.
2. Q waves in lead V_1 alone are ignored unless there are other abnormalities in precordial leads.
3. Q waves in lead III alone are ignored unless there are abnormalities in other inferior leads (for example, aVF or II, or both). To be significant, Q waves in inferior leads III and aVF must be wider or deeper, or both, than Q waves in anterior leads.
4. Q waves together with ST segment or T wave abnormalities in the same lead tend to be more reliable for the diagnosis of myocardial infarction than Q waves without such ST-T abnormalities.
5. Q waves in the presence of LBBB or other major IVCDs are usually not significant and are generally ignored. This does not apply to RBBB, in which Q waves have their usual significance. Q waves in the presence of LVH are less reliable for the diagnosis of myocardial infarction, and the ECG must be examined very carefully for the presence of diminutive R waves, which usually indicate that no infarction is present.
6. The most commonly used single criterion for a Q wave significant for myocardial infarction is duration (width) ≥ 0.04 second or amplitude (depth) $\geq$ one-fourth of the R wave in the same lead.

For *diaphragmatic myocardial infarction (DMI)*, highly specific criteria for significant Q waves include duration ≥ 0.04 second, depth ≥ 5 mm, or depth $\geq$ one-third of R wave amplitude in leads II, III *and* aVF (often with T wave inversions in those same leads). Moderately specific criteria for DMI include Q waves ≥ 0.04-second duration and depth greater than one-fourth of the R wave amplitude in lead II *or* aVF. Less specific criteria for DMI include Q waves ≥ 0.03 second and of any depth in lead II alone or Q waves ≥ 0.04 second or ≥ 5 mm deep in lead aVF alone.

Q waves occurring solely in lead III are quite unreliable; they often vary greatly in duration and depth or even disappear entirely with deep inspiration or other maneuvers that shift the position of the heart within the chest. A Q wave in lead III alone, even if ≥ 0.04-second duration or ≥ 5 mm deep, should not be considered evidence of DMI unless a Q wave ≥ 1 mm is also present in lead aVF. Even this combination, which, according to some classifications, would permit a diagnosis of possible DMI, is only suggestive of DMI. Significant Q waves also should be present in lead aVF or, for even more certainty, in lead aVF *and* lead II before DMI is diagnosed from the ECG.

For *anterior myocardial infarction (AMI)*, the most specific Q wave criteria include Q wave or QS complex ≥0.03-second duration and depth ≥one-third of the R wave height in any of leads I and V_2 through V_6, or Q wave duration ≥0.03 second in any two precordial leads. A bit less specific, but still highly accurate, is the generally accepted criterion of Q wave duration ≥0.04 second or depth more than one-fourth of the corresponding R wave amplitude in lead I or V_2 through V_6 (or aVL with an R wave ≥3 mm in that lead).

Less specific criteria include Q wave >0.03-second duration with depth ≥one-third of the corresponding R wave amplitude in leads V_2 through V_6. Even a diminutive Q wave may be significant in lead V_2 or V_3 if the lead has a right ventricular configuration, that is, a Q wave, then a small R wave, and a larger S wave (Atlas ECG 7-2). Ordinarily, there should be no Q waves whatever in leads V_2 and V_3 unless the heart is rotated counterclockwise and lead V_2 or V_3 is recorded over the left ventricle with its (normal) tiny septal Q wave (Atlas ECG 7-3).

Another less specific criterion for AMI is the pattern often termed "poor R wave progression." R waves, usually small in leads V_1 and V_2, normally increase in amplitude in leads moving to the left across the chest (V_1 through V_5), for the succeeding precordial leads lie over the bulk of the left ventricle, which should produce substantial R waves. In poor R wave progression, precordial R waves do not increase in amplitude moving from V_1 to V_2 to V_3 and on to the left.

Quite specific for the diagnosis of AMI is actual decrease of the R wave in leads moving to the left; that is, the R wave in V_2 might be 5 mm and the R wave in V_3, which should be taller than in V_2, may decrease to 2 mm — particularly if there are associated T wave inversions in these leads. Also quite specific for AMI is a QS complex — that is, no R wave whatever — in lead V_2, V_3 or V_4, as long as the succeeding lead to the right does have an R wave.

Much less specific is an R wave of 1 or 2 mm that does not change much in leads V_2, V_3 and V_4. If the T waves are upright in these leads, the diagnosis of AMI is unlikely and the significance of the diagnosis "poor R wave progression" is uncertain. Such a situation may arise with clockwise rotation of the heart or with noncardiac problems such as pericardial or pleural effusion, which causes low R wave voltage.

Although these "rules" appear quite complex, it should be emphasized that the average ECG reader is well served by remembering the criteria for significant Q waves first cited in this section: *a "significant" Q wave indicating likely myocardial infarction is ≥0.04 second in duration or has a depth ≥one-fourth of the corresponding R wave amplitude, or both.*

The differential diagnosis of "significant" Q waves is very brief — myocardial infarction or idiopathic hypertrophic subaortic stenosis (IHSS). The latter is an unusual condition that illustrates some of the points regarding Q wave pathogenesis made previously. As mentioned, a small Q wave in left ventricular leads such as I, aVL, V_5 or V_6 is normal and is a result of physiologic depolarization of the interventricular septum from left to right. In IHSS, the septum is hypertrophied; thus, septal forces have increased amplitude and also require a longer time to traverse the larger muscle mass of the abnormal septum. So, Q waves in IHSS may exceed 0.04 second in duration and one-fourth of the R wave in amplitude and still be septal

Q waves rather than indicative of myocardial infarction (Plate 21, bottom; Atlas ECG 7-4).

Substantial LVH is often present in IHSS. This LVH, together with T wave abnormalities that may be marked and bizarre, may be a clue to the electrocardiographer that large Q waves are due to IHSS rather than myocardial infarction. The clinical setting, for example, a harsh systolic murmur at the left sternal border that increases with the Valsalva maneuver, aids in clarifying the diagnosis.

Effects of Myocardial Ischemia, Injury, and Infarction on the ECG

Myocardial infarction, the process leading to actual necrosis of tissue, produces Q waves if necrosis involves the entire thickness of the ventricular wall. If only a portion of the wall — usually the more vulnerable subendocardial layer — is damaged, Q waves do not develop and ST segments and T waves are abnormal.

Plate 22 summarizes the electrocardiographic changes seen in myocardial ischemia, which causes the least severe interference with myocardial perfusion and metabolism and which generally affects only the subendocardial portion of the myocardium. Myocardial ischemia alone causes depression of the ST segment, often with associated T wave inversion — electrocardiographic changes that are due to abnormalities of repolarization. Plate 22 shows a zone of ischemia at the border of an infarcted and injured area, but myocardial ischemia often occurs in the absence of either injury or infarction. Since the main coronary arteries are located on the outside (epicardial) surface of the heart, with branches traversing the myocardium to supply the inner muscle layers, it is not surprising that the distant subendocardium is most vulnerable to ischemia. Ischemia and its associated ST segment and T wave changes may come and go very quickly, for example, during an anginal attack or during exercise stress testing. Ischemia also may be present at the border of a myocardial infarction, as in Plate 22, and may disappear more gradually as healing proceeds.

Elevation of the ST segment has been described as being due to myocardial "injury," shown in Plate 22 as a zone closer to the irreversibly damaged central area of a myocardial infarction. (ST segment elevation may also be termed "current of injury.") When ST elevation occurs in the course of acute myocardial infarction, the myocardial injury is often severe and progressive. Necrosis commonly develops in areas where ST segment elevation was present in the early stages of the infarction. However, the pathophysiologic change represented by ST segment elevation is not always progressive and irreversible. For example, in vasospastic angina (page 65), marked ST segment elevation can appear and disappear within a few minutes and leave no permanent sequelae.

Radionuclide studies of myocardial perfusion indicate that ST segment *depression* represents mild to moderate deprivation of flow primarily affecting the subendocardial layers of myocardium, whereas ST segment *elevation* associated with the severe transmural deprivation of flow affects subepicardial as well as subendocardial layers of myocardium. Prolonged, severe, and extensive deprivation of flow may lead to necrosis, as in myocardial infarction; if it is quickly reversed, there may be no sequelae and no tissue injury.

Plate 22

Effects of Myocardial Ischemia, Injury, and Infarction on ECG

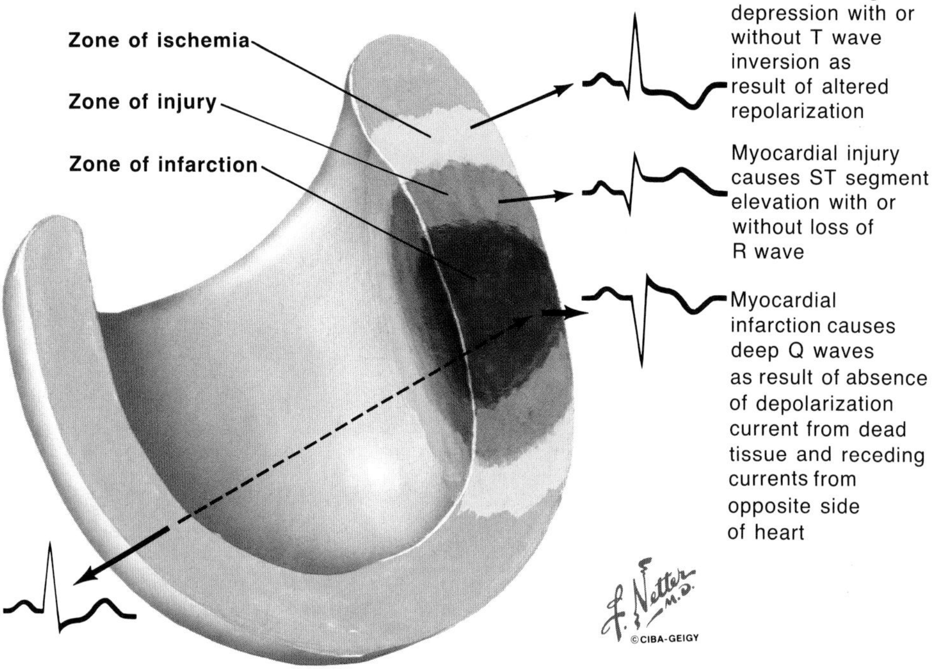

Zone of ischemia

Zone of injury

Zone of infarction

Myocardial ischemia causes ST segment depression with or without T wave inversion as result of altered repolarization

Myocardial injury causes ST segment elevation with or without loss of R wave

Myocardial infarction causes deep Q waves as result of absence of depolarization current from dead tissue and receding currents from opposite side of heart

Plate 22 also depicts a zone of infarction that, if transmural, causes Q waves because the dead myocardium under the given electrode(s) generates no electrical activity. Thus, most electrical forces, especially those emanating from the opposite wall of the heart, are moving away from the electrode and generate a negative ECG deflection (the Q wave).

Plate 23 details progressive stages of the pathologic and electrocardiographic manifestations of acute myocardial infarction.

Transmural infarction. In transmural infarction (Plate 23, top panel), ST segment elevation, sometimes with increased amplitude and peaking of the T waves, or prolongation of the QT interval is the first electrocardiographic manifestation. Little if any myocardial tissue has died, and thus the R wave remains largely intact (Plate 23, top panel, second diagram; Atlas ECG 7-5; see also ECG 7-8). Within several hours after the onset of acute myocardial infarction, some myocardial cells begin to die, and the R wave amplitude diminishes while Q wave depth or duration may increase. Peaked or high-amplitude T waves generally disappear, whereas ST segment elevation usually persists and may be very prominent (Plate 23, top panel, third diagram; see also Atlas ECG 7-9).

Within 2 days after the onset of infarction, most jeopardized tissue has died, the R wave has disappeared, and a significant Q wave is present. ST segments return toward the baseline and T wave inversion begins (Plate 23, top panel, fourth diagram; Atlas ECGs 7-6 and 7-7). After several days, transmural infarction is complete and little or no injured or ischemic tissue remains, as all cells have either died or recovered. At this point,

ST segments are generally at the baseline and T wave inversions are progressing (Plate 23, top panel, fifth diagram). Several weeks or months after infarction, infarcted tissue is replaced by fibrous tissue, often with thinning and sometimes aneurysmal dilatation of the necrotic portion of the ventricular wall.

At times, islands of myocardial tissue within the infarcted area that were electrically silent during the acute period of the infarction recover some electrical activity. If this occurs, some R waves may return, although the significant Q wave representing transmural infarction usually persists. If a ventricular aneurysm of significant size develops, ST segments may remain elevated (page 69). T waves may remain inverted for years, may return to baseline, or may become upright again after variable periods of time (Plate 23, top panel, sixth diagram; see also Atlas ECG 7-10).

Subendocardial infarction. The early stages of subendocardial infarction are characterized by depressed or elevated ST segments with variable T wave abnormalities (Plate 23, bottom panel, second diagram). Although some tissue dies, the amount of necrosis is usually less than in transmural infarction, and necrosis does not extend through to the epicardial wall. Thus, there is always electrically active tissue under any electrocardiographic electrode, and significant Q waves by definition do not develop. The R wave amplitude may be somewhat diminished; however, R waves persist and ST segments are depressed or elevated, depending on whether ischemia is subendocardial or transmural, the former condition being much more common.

Once jeopardized tissue has either died or recovered so that ischemia is no longer present, ST segments usually return to baseline; T wave abnormalities — often T wave inversions — may persist (Plate 23, bottom panel, third diagram). Healing occurs after several weeks or months; thinning and aneurysmal dilatation of the ventricular wall are uncommon in subendocardial infarction. ST segment depressions and T wave inversions may persist or may return to normal (Plate 23, bottom panel, fourth diagram).

As noted previously in other contexts, many descriptive terms persist in electrocardiography with less than perfect anatomic validation. The previous discussion of transmural and subendocardial infarctions is one prominent example. Sophisticated new diagnostic techniques and careful clinical-pathologic correlations indicate that electrocardiographic Q wave and non-Q wave patterns are not always synonymous with transmural and subendocardial infarctions, respectively. It has been suggested that the type of infarction described in Plate 23, top panel, be termed a "Q wave infarction," without implications that this electrocardiographic pattern always denotes transmural damage, and the infarction described in Plate 23, bottom panel, be called "non-Q wave infarction," without implication that this electrocardiographic pattern always represents less than transmural or subendocardial damages. Of interest is the fact that although electrocardiographic patterns are admittedly imprecise in their anatomic implications, they have great significance: Q wave infarctions are generally larger, have a higher incidence of early complications like pulmonary edema and cardiogenic shock, and are far more likely to be associated with a complete thrombotic occlusion of the coronary artery supplying the infarcted area. Despite these caveats, Q wave infarctions *are* more likely to represent transmural damage and, among other corollaries of that fact, are less likely to show improvement of regional

Plate 23

Progressive Stages and Electrocardiographic

Transmural Infarction

Before coronary occlusion — Onset and first several hours — First day

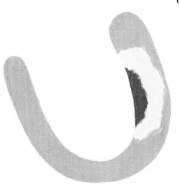
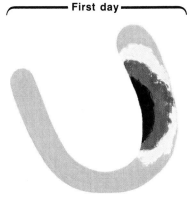

Heart muscle normal

Subendocardial injury and myocardial ischemia. No cell death (infarction) yet

Ischemia and injury extend to epicardial surface. Subendo-cardial muscle dying in area of most severe injury

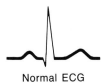
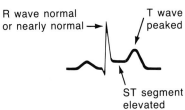

R wave normal or nearly normal →

T wave peaked

Normal ECG

ST segment elevated

R wave amplitude diminishing

ST elevation more marked

Subendocardial Infarction

Before infarction — First few hours

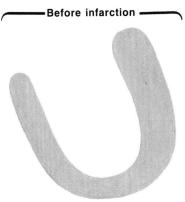
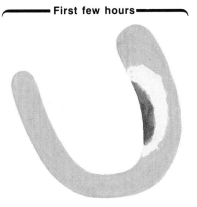

Heart muscle normal

Subendocardial muscle ischemic and injured but not dead

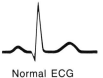

Normal ECG

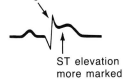

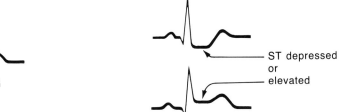

ST depressed or elevated

F. Netter
©CIBA-GEIGY

Manifestations of Myocardial Infarction

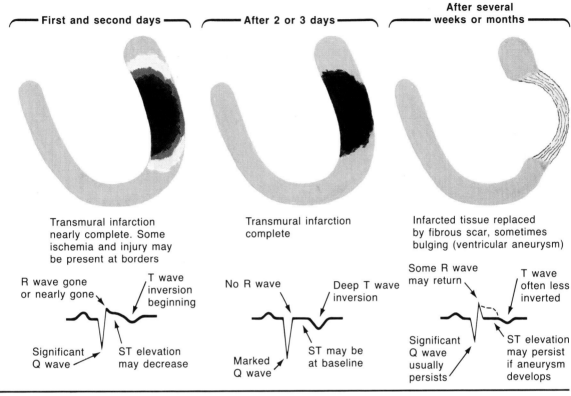

First and second days

Transmural infarction nearly complete. Some ischemia and injury may be present at borders

R wave gone or nearly gone

T wave inversion beginning

Significant Q wave

ST elevation may decrease

After 2 or 3 days

Transmural infarction complete

No R wave

Deep T wave inversion

Marked Q wave

ST may be at baseline

After several weeks or months

Infarcted tissue replaced by fibrous scar, sometimes bulging (ventricular aneurysm)

Some R wave may return

T wave often less inverted

Significant Q wave usually persists

ST elevation may persist if aneurysm develops

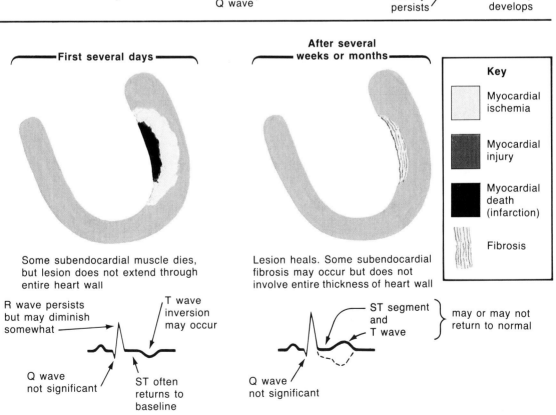

First several days

Some subendocardial muscle dies, but lesion does not extend through entire heart wall

R wave persists but may diminish somewhat

T wave inversion may occur

Q wave not significant

ST often returns to baseline

After several weeks or months

Lesion heals. Some subendocardial fibrosis may occur but does not involve entire thickness of heart wall

ST segment and T wave } may or may not return to normal

Q wave not significant

Key

Myocardial ischemia

Myocardial injury

Myocardial death (infarction)

Fibrosis

59

myocardial function after successful coronary bypass surgery to the area of Q wave damage.

In contrast, non-Q wave infarctions are, in general, smaller, associated with fewer early hemodynamic complications, and have a much lower incidence of coronary thrombosis and total occlusion of the coronary artery supplying the infarction. However, the rate of reinfarction and sudden death within a few months after the original non-Q wave infarction is disturbingly high, perhaps as a subtotal coronary occlusion becomes total or as ischemic but not dead tissue at the borders of nontransmural damage goes on to infarction. Non-Q wave infarctions now cause great concern with regard to short-term follow-up, and it is the ECG — not more sophisticated tests — that seems to best identify this interesting group of patients.

Localization of Myocardial Infarctions and Ischemia

Occlusive disease of the left anterior descending coronary artery or its branches produces pathologic and electrocardiographic changes in the anterior myocardial wall. Lead I and the precordial leads reveal anterior infarction or ischemia. Plate 24, top panel, shows a large transmural anterior myocardial infarction caused by occlusion of the proximal left anterior descending coronary artery. A large area of the anterior wall has become necrotic; the ECG shows a significant Q wave in lead I, QS complexes with total loss of R wave and T wave inversion in leads V_1 through V_4, and some loss of R wave with T wave flattening or inversion extending laterally to leads V_5 and V_6. Atlas ECGs 7-5 through 7-7 show another anterior myocardial infarction, with QS complexes developing only in leads V_1 and V_2 but with more widespread anterior T wave abnormalities. Anterior wall ischemia or subendocardial infarction would be seen in the same leads, but in this case, ST segment and T wave abnormalities would be prominent and the Q waves or major R wave abnormalities would not occur.

An infarction of the anterolateral wall is depicted in Plate 24, bottom panel. Such an infarction might result from occlusion of the left circumflex coronary artery; the marginal (sometimes termed "obtuse marginal") vessel, which is often a large and important branch of the circumflex; or a large diagonal branch of the left anterior descending coronary artery. Since coronary anatomy and the size and importance of the coronary arteries vary among different persons, any or all of the vessels mentioned might supply the lateral wall of the left ventricle. In *transmural anterolateral infarction*, significant Q waves occur in leads I, aVL, and perhaps V_5 or V_6, or both, often with ST segment abnormalities or T wave inversions in those leads. Anterolateral ischemia or subendocardial infarction produces ST segment and T wave changes in leads I, aVL, and perhaps V_5 and V_6, but no Q waves in those leads.

The large inferior surface of the heart rests on the diaphragm; thus, infarction or ischemia in this location may be termed "inferior" or "diaphragmatic." In most persons, the diaphragmatic wall of the heart is supplied by the right coronary artery and its distal tributaries, the posterior descending artery and posterolateral branches. This common pattern of coronary anatomy is called *right-dominant* coronary circulation. When the diaphragmatic wall is supplied by the right coronary artery, the circumflex is often small, and it may be diminutive beyond the obtuse marginal branch.

In some persons, however, the circumflex is the large vessel, continuing around to the diaphragmatic surface in the groove between the left atrium and the left ventricle and giving off the posterior descending artery. In this case, the right coronary artery is smaller and may be diminutive. When the diaphragmatic wall is supplied by the distal left circumflex coronary artery, the coronary circulation is said to be *left dominant*.

In still other persons, both right coronary and left circumflex arteries are of good size, and both continue around to the rear of the heart in their respective atrioventricular grooves to jointly supply the posterior descending and other posterior arteries. This is known as *balanced* or *codominant* coronary circulation.

Plate 25, top panel, depicts the more common situation, in which occlusion of the right coronary artery has caused a transmural diaphragmatic infarction. This produces significant Q waves with T wave inversions in leads II, III and aVF, the leads that reflect electrical activity of the inferior wall (Atlas ECGs 7-8 through 7-10). A diaphragmatic infarction or ischemia often extends to the lateral wall, in which case changes are also seen in lead V_5 or V_6 (as in Plate 25). It is also not uncommon for a diaphragmatic infarction or ischemia to extend to the true posterior surface of the heart (Atlas ECG 7-11). Diaphragmatic ischemia or subendocardial infarction produces ST segment and T wave changes without Q wave or R wave abnormalities in leads II, III and aVF.

The true posterior, as opposed to the inferior, surface of the heart is relatively small and may be supplied by either the distal left circumflex or the distal right coronary artery or branches thereof. A true posterior infarction is diagnosed much less often than infarction of other areas of the heart. This is partially because the posterior surface is relatively small and has the potential for blood supply from either the distal right or the distal circumflex system. However, the main reason for the infrequent recognition of true posterior disease is the fact that no leads of the standard ECG face the true posterior surface of the heart. Thus, abnormalities of the true posterior wall must be diagnosed indirectly by the reciprocal changes they produce on the opposite surface, that is, reciprocal changes on the anterior wall of the heart, as seen in lead V_1.

Q waves or loss of R waves posteriorly would be expected in transmural infarction of the posterior surface. (Q waves may actually be seen if the electrocardiographer has the patient swallow an ECG lead and positions the lead in the esophagus directly facing the posterior wall of the heart!) The reciprocal of a loss of R wave voltage posteriorly is a gain in voltage in the anterior leads, diagnosed as increased R wave voltage in lead V_1. The reciprocal of posterior T wave inversion is an upright T wave in the anterior lead V_1. Plate 25, bottom panel, shows the subtle changes of a true posterior myocardial infarction, characterized by increased anterior R wave voltage (R wave ≥ 0.04-second duration with amplitude greater than that of the S wave in lead V_1) and upright T wave in lead V_1 (Atlas ECG 7-11). (See Table 1 for the differential diagnosis of a tall R wave in lead V_1, which includes right ventricular hypertrophy and counterclockwise rotation [page 43, Atlas ECG 7-12]). True posterior infarction is easily missed if the R wave voltage in lead V_1 is not markedly increased, but a high index of

Plate 24

Localization of Myocardial Infarcts

Anterior infarct

Occlusion of proximal left anterior descending coronary artery

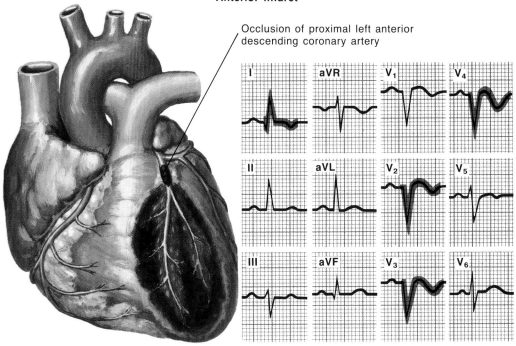

Significant Q waves and T wave inversions in leads I, V_2, V_3 and V_4

Anterolateral infarct

Occlusion of
left circumflex coronary artery,
marginal branch of left circumflex artery, or
diagonal branch of left anterior descending artery

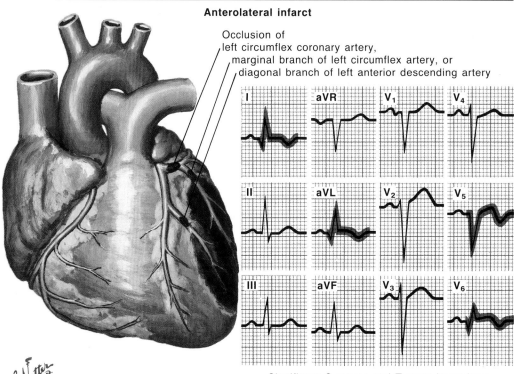

Significant Q waves and T wave inversions in leads I, aVL, V_5 and V_6

Plate 25

Localization of Myocardial Infarcts (continued)

Diaphragmatic or inferior infarct

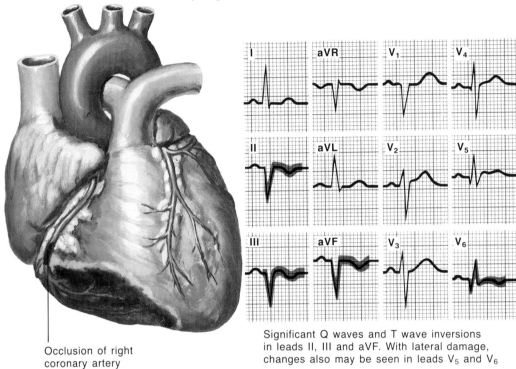

Occlusion of right coronary artery

Significant Q waves and T wave inversions in leads II, III and aVF. With lateral damage, changes also may be seen in leads V_5 and V_6

True posterior infarct

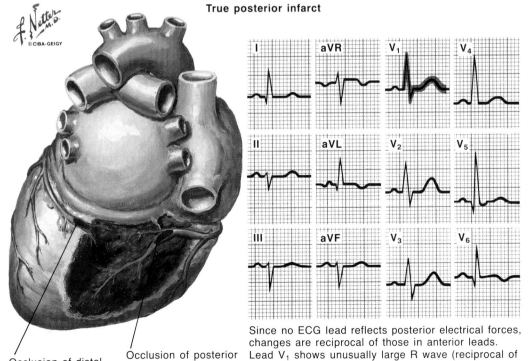

Occlusion of distal circumflex artery or Occlusion of posterior descending or distal right coronary arteries

Since no ECG lead reflects posterior electrical forces, changes are reciprocal of those in anterior leads. Lead V_1 shows unusually large R wave (reciprocal of posterior Q wave) and upright T wave (reciprocal of posterior T wave inversion)

suspicion for posterior involvement is necessary in cases of diaphragmatic or diaphragmatic and lateral infarction, since the same diseased right or distal circumflex coronary artery often supplies both diaphragmatic and posterior surfaces.

One final anatomic "location" of myocardial infarction is subendocardial. Strictly speaking, any nontransmural infarction is subendocardial; this is diagnosed from the clinical history, ST segment and T wave changes without development of Q waves, and elevation of cardiac enzymes in the serum (Plate 23, bottom panel). A variant often singled out is *widespread* subendocardial infarction, in which deep, symmetrical T wave inversions develop in all or nearly all leads except aVR (Atlas ECG 7-13). The resulting infarction is pathologically characterized by necrosis of a large portion of the entire subendocardial layer of the left ventricle, which may better be related to a *generalized* problem of poor subendocardial perfusion (for example, a period of hypotension occurring during general anesthesia) rather than to a *local* atherosclerotic lesion in the distribution of a narrowed coronary artery. It would be better to use the term "widespread subendocardial" to refer specifically to this type of infarction and to speak of the smaller, non-Q wave infarction in the territory of one coronary artery as "anterior nontransmural" or "inferior nontransmural." However, in everyday practice, both types of infarction are confusingly termed simply "subendocardial," and the reader must consult the actual ECG to differentiate between the two.

8 ST SEGMENT AND T WAVE ABNORMALITIES

ST Segment Elevations

The most common cause of ST segment elevation is the current of injury, although as previously noted, this is probably just a manifestation of intense transmural myocardial ischemia. Most often caused by occlusion of a large coronary artery (Plate 26, top panel; Atlas ECGs 7-5 and 7-8), intense transmural ischemia is frequently seen in the early stages of acute myocardial infarction. Although the pathophysiology of ST segment elevation is not certain, it is known that intracellular potassium leaks from injured tissue. The resting potential of myocardial cells depends on the ratio of intracellular to extracellular potassium, and the baseline of the ECG (arbitrarily set in electrical diastole, during the interval from the end of the preceding T wave to the next P wave) is related to the resting potential of the myocardial cells. Thus, leakage of potassium from injured tissue with reduction of intracellular potassium lowers the baseline of the ECG.

Depolarization (the QRS complex) and repolarization (the ST segment and the T wave) are much less affected by the ionic ratio that sets the level of the baseline during electrical diastole. Since the ECG reader has no absolute standard for the baseline of the ECG and simply assumes that it is the constant from which all other deflections are measured, lowering of the baseline because of myocardial cell injury and consequent potassium loss, with no change in the electrical potential during ST segment and T wave inscription, gives the mistaken impression that the ST segment and T wave are elevated.

If intense transmural ischemia is caused by atherosclerotic occlusion or thrombosis of a major coronary artery, or both, myocardial infarction ensues, tissue becomes necrotic, potassium leak ceases, and the baseline returns to normal. ST segment elevation disappears and the other abnormalities of myocardial infarction — loss of R wave, development of significant Q wave, and T wave inversion — are seen (Plate 26, top panel; Atlas ECGs 7-10 and 7-11).

Another cause of intense transmural myocardial ischemia is coronary vasospasm (Plate 26, bottom panel). Vasospasm is the cause of Prinzmetal's (variant) angina, an unusual form of angina in which chest pain is not related to exertion, may be associated with major arrhythmias, and often comes and goes quickly many times a day without obvious precipitating factors.

Electrocardiographically, Prinzmetal's angina with ST segment elevation cannot be differentiated from the current of injury seen in the early stages of acute myocardial infarction. Patients with chest pain and ST segment elevation are usually admitted to the hospital, where testing generally establishes the diagnosis. Either progressive electrocardiographic changes and elevation of serum enzymes such as creatine kinase establish the cause of ST segment elevation as acute myocardial infarction, or recurrent transient attacks of pain and ST segment elevation suggest the diagnosis of Prinzmetal's angina, which can be confirmed angiographically if necessary. Recent evidence suggests that coronary vasospasm also occurs in patients without typical Prinzmetal's angina; transient ST segment elevation in such patients can be very confusing but should suggest the diagnosis of coronary vasospasm.

Acute pericarditis also causes ST segment elevation. Since pericarditis is also associated with chest pain, patients with acute pericarditis are often hospitalized for suspected acute myocardial infarction. There are, however, several differentiating features. First, patients with pericarditis often are younger, lack coronary risk factors, and are not suspected of having atherosclerotic coronary artery disease. Second, the pain of pericarditis is frequently relieved by sitting upright and leaning forward, and may be pleuritic (worse with inspiration). The pain may persist for hours or even days, longer than in most cases of myocardial infarction. With the characteristic clinical history, particularly if a pericardial friction rub is heard on physical examination, the diagnosis of pericarditis is not difficult. Of great importance electrocardiographically is the fact that pericarditis is usually a generalized pathologic process. Thus, the ST segment elevation of acute pericarditis may be seen in anterior, lateral, diaphragmatic, and other areas of the heart.

Generalized ST segment elevation as depicted in Plate 27, bottom left, and Atlas ECG 8-1 is unrelated to the anatomic distribution of the coronary arteries. Atherosclerotic occlusive disease of the left anterior descending coronary artery should produce anterior changes, that of the left circumflex coronary artery should produce lateral changes, and that of the right coronary artery should produce inferior changes. The fact that electrocardiographic changes are seen in so many different anatomic areas implies that the abnormality is not related to the coronary arteries.

There are many different types of acute pericarditis, including the relatively common idiopathic benign pericarditis that is often of viral origin.

Plate 26

ST Segment Elevations

Acute myocardial injury

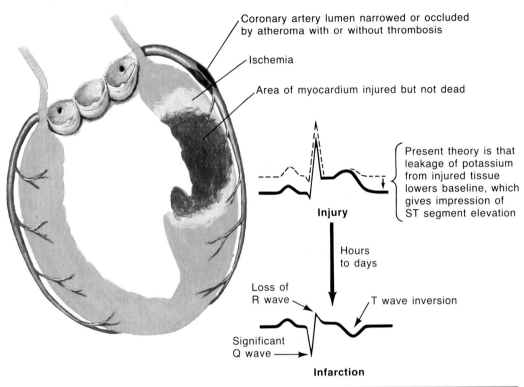

Coronary artery lumen narrowed or occluded by atheroma with or without thrombosis

Ischemia

Area of myocardium injured but not dead

Injury

Present theory is that leakage of potassium from injured tissue lowers baseline, which gives impression of ST segment elevation

Hours to days

Loss of R wave

T wave inversion

Significant Q wave

Infarction

Vasospasm with intense transmural myocardial ischemia (often Prinzmetal's [variant] angina)

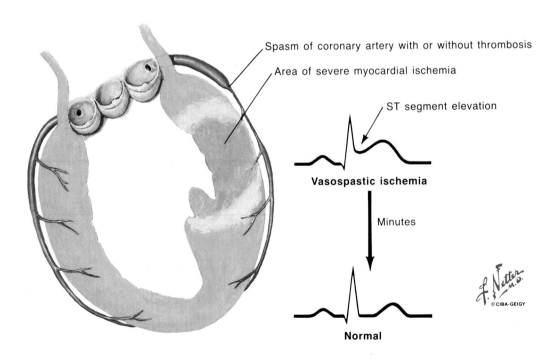

Spasm of coronary artery with or without thrombosis

Area of severe myocardial ischemia

ST segment elevation

Vasospastic ischemia

Minutes

Normal

©CIBA-GEIGY

Plate 27

ST Segment Elevations (continued)

Pericarditis

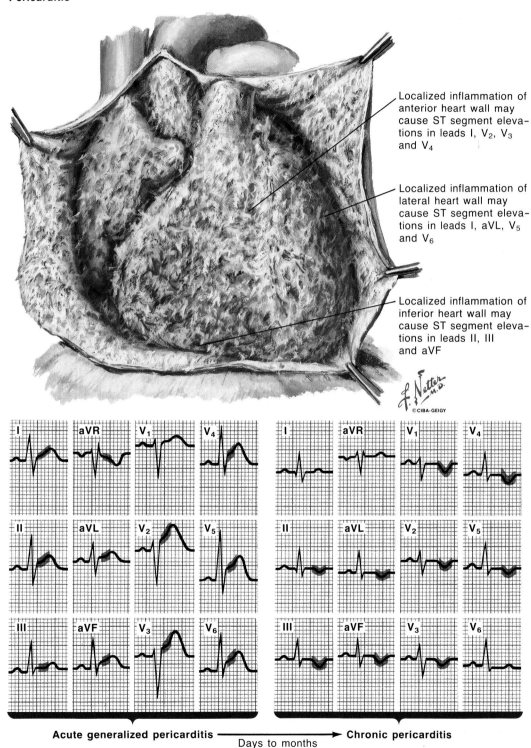

Localized inflammation of anterior heart wall may cause ST segment elevations in leads I, V_2, V_3 and V_4

Localized inflammation of lateral heart wall may cause ST segment elevations in leads I, aVL, V_5 and V_6

Localized inflammation of inferior heart wall may cause ST segment elevations in leads II, III and aVF

Acute generalized pericarditis ————————→ **Chronic pericarditis**

Days to months

ST segment elevations in many leads

ST segment elevations resolved. Widespread T wave inversions present

Plate 28

ST Segment Elevations (continued)

Ventricular aneurysm

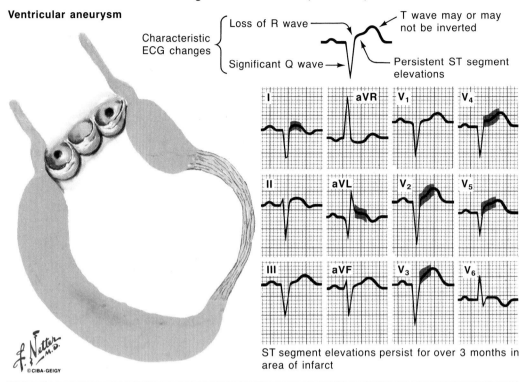

Characteristic ECG changes:
- Loss of R wave
- Significant Q wave
- T wave may or may not be inverted
- Persistent ST segment elevations

ST segment elevations persist for over 3 months in area of infarct

---

Early repolarization (normal variant often seen in young people)

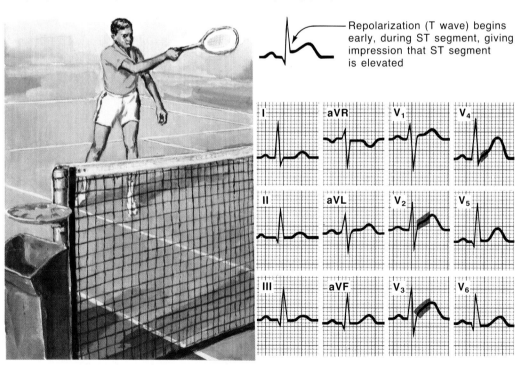

Repolarization (T wave) begins early, during ST segment, giving impression that ST segment is elevated

Asymptomatic young person, usually with no suspicion of heart disease

ST segment elevations usually most evident in leads V_2, V_3 and V_4, without other ECG abnormalities

Some types of pericarditis are not so benign, such as uremic, bacterial, or tuberculous pericarditis, the pericarditis of systemic lupus erythematosus or other collagen diseases, and the pericarditis caused by malignant disease. With time, the ST segment elevations of acute pericarditis generally return to baseline, often to be replaced by widespread T wave inversions (Plate 27, bottom right; Atlas ECG 8-2). If pericardial effusion develops, QRS voltage declines notably, which may be a valuable aid in the diagnosis of the potentially life-threatening pericardial tamponade.

A rare electrocardiographic finding quite specific for the diagnosis of pericardial effusion is electrical alternans, that is, alternating higher and lower amplitude of electrocardiographic waves — either the QRS complex alone or, sometimes, the entire P-QRS-T complex. Echocardiographic investigations have shown that major shifts of the heart as it swings excessively in the fluid in the pericardial sac cause beat-to-beat changes in the electrical axis and thus corresponding changes in amplitude of ECG waves, producing electrical alternans.

ST segment elevations also often occur with ventricular aneurysm, which sometimes results from acute myocardial infarction (Plate 28, top panel; Atlas ECG 7-7). A ventricular aneurysm is diagnosed from the ECG when ST segment elevation persists for some time after recovery from the acute infarction. (The time period may vary, but most authorities cite 3 months.) The infarction is almost always obvious, with significant Q waves in the leads with ST segment elevations. Unfortunately, ST segment elevation is estimated to be present in only about one-third of aneurysms, and thus is not a very sensitive clue to ventricular aneurysm.

One final cause of ST segment elevation is a normal variant termed "early repolarization" (Plate 28, bottom; Atlas ECG 8-3). In some perfectly normal persons — particularly those under age 30, males, and blacks — the T wave representing repolarization of the myocardium begins during the ST segment, giving the impression that the ST segment is elevated. This finding is most common in right precordial leads such as V_2 and V_3, but it may be seen in other leads. The ST elevation of early repolarization may be quite marked, 1 to 3 mm or more. The contour of the ST segment (concave upward, convex upward, and so forth) cannot reliably be differentiated from myocardial injury, pericarditis, or other conditions causing ST segment elevation.

Early repolarization is seen so often in the normal population that it is valuable to obtain one baseline ECG in most young people before they reach the age when coronary artery disease is prevalent. Although ST segment elevation can be presumed to be the normal variant of early repolarization in a 21-year-old asymptomatic athlete having a routine ECG, ST elevations in a 45-year-old male who complains of chest pain might indicate a major problem. It is sometimes necessary to admit such patients to the hospital because of suspicion of myocardial infarction; however, if a prior ECG is available showing that early repolarization was present in the past, such confusion can often be avoided.

ST Segment Depressions

A common and important cause of ST segment depression is myocardial ischemia. Although ST segment depressions with or without T wave abnormalities can be chronic, these depressions are much more commonly transient and temporally associated with acute myocardial ischemia. A familiar example of such transient myocardial ischemia is that induced by having the patient perform physical exercise, generally either walking on a treadmill or pedaling a bicycle.

Plate 29, left panel, depicts the myocardium and the ECG before exercise. Although a coronary artery is significantly narrowed, sufficient blood reaches the resting myocardium so that no ischemia is present and the ECG is normal. As the patient performs physical exercise, heart rate and myocardial work increase, but coronary artery stenosis limits the increase of flow needed to meet the exercise-induced increase in myocardial oxygen demand. When ischemia develops, the patient often feels anginal chest pain. Myocardial contractility generally decreases (either a global decline in function or, more commonly, a regional decline in contraction in the ischemic area), and ST segment depressions are seen on the ECG in the ischemic area (Plate 29, right panel; Atlas ECGs 8-4A and B).

The exercise stress test has been well standardized as to the implications of various electrocardiographic findings. For a reasonably certain diagnosis of ischemia, sufficient exercise must be performed to increase the heart rate (an indirect but surprisingly useful measure of myocardial oxygen needs) to at least 85% of the maximum achievable heart rate for that patient. (The maximum heart rate varies according to age and sex, but it can be approximated from the formula: maximum heart rate = 220 minus one-half of age.)

Several types of ST segment depressions are associated with myocardial ischemia (Plate 30). One widely accepted criterion for "significant" ST segment depression is J point depression ≥1 mm (0.10 mv) and ST segment depression ≥1 mm from 0.06 to 0.08 second (60 to 80 msec) after the J point. (The J point is that point at which the QRS complex ends and the ST segment begins. At times, the R wave or S wave ends abruptly, but sometimes, the slope merely changes as the QRS complex merges into the ST segment.)

Some authorities measure ST depression at a single point, either 0.06 or 0.08 second after the end of the QRS, while others require that the ST segment remain depressed for at least 0.02 to 0.04 second at some time after the end of the QRS complex. It is easy to remember these complicated "rules" by using a simplified version of the American Heart Association criterion: ST segment depression ≥1 mm at 0.08 second (two small vertically ruled boxes) after the end of the QRS complex usually indicates ischemia.

The ST depressions of myocardial ischemia have been subclassified according to their slope. Many electrocardiographers speak of "upsloping," "horizontal," and "downsloping" ST segment depressions, but no matter which way the ST segment is sloping, a significant depression must meet the criterion of ≥1-mm depression 0.08 second after the end of the QRS (Plate 30). Downsloping ST segment depression is the most specific for myocardial ischemia, horizontal depression is of intermediate specificity, and upsloping depression is the least specific.

It must be recognized that any electrocardiographic criterion for significance is arbitrary and is a balance of the desired sensitivity and specificity. A very strict criterion for significant ST depression, for example, 2 mm of downsloping ST segment depression, would be highly specific, permitting a diagnosis of myocardial ischemia that could be confirmed by coronary

Plate 29

ST Segment Depressions

Myocardial ischemia, demonstrated by stress test

At rest

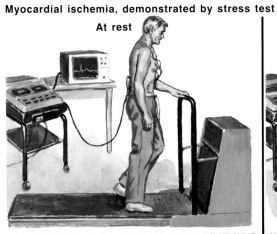

Exercise

Incline and speed
of treadmill
progressively
increased

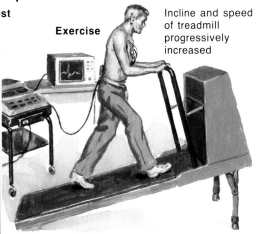

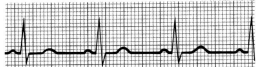

Heart rate normal for resting state

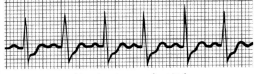

Heart rate accelerated

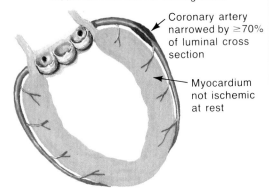

Coronary artery
narrowed by ≥70%
of luminal cross
section

Myocardium
not ischemic
at rest

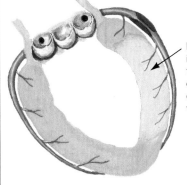

Myocardium
ischemic due
to increased
demand for
coronary flow
with exercise

©CIBA-GEIGY

Normal ECG. No ST
segment depressions

ST segment depressions in
leads overlying ischemic zone

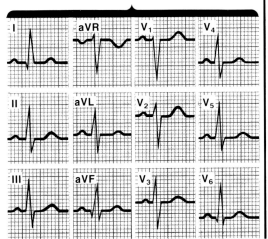

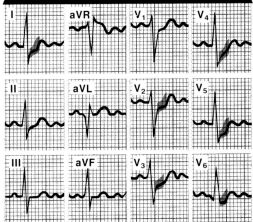

Plate 30

Types of ST Segment Depressions

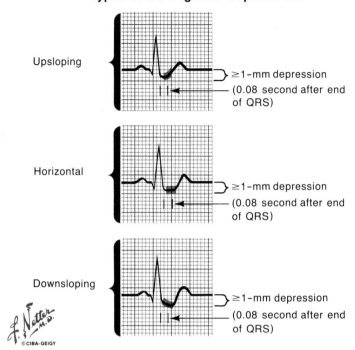

Upsloping

≥1-mm depression
(0.08 second after end of QRS)

Horizontal

≥1-mm depression
(0.08 second after end of QRS)

Downsloping

≥1-mm depression
(0.08 second after end of QRS)

angiography in most cases. There would be very few false-positive results of stress tests if such a standard were used. However, such a strict criterion would be relatively insensitive and would fail to detect many cases of lesser degrees of myocardial ischemia and thus lesser changes on the stress ECG.

On the other hand, if one were to employ the criterion of 0.50 mm of ST segment depression with a slope in any direction, this would detect the vast majority of cases of myocardial ischemia but would be far too sensitive and yield false-positive results in many patients with only minor electrocardiographic changes not associated with significant coronary artery disease or myocardial ischemia. This would lead to overdiagnosis of ischemic heart disease and to unnecessary further studies such as radionuclide stress testing or coronary angiography to prove that the minor ST segment depression was not caused by myocardial ischemia.

To strike a balance between specificity and sensitivity, the 1-mm criterion has been generally accepted. However, no diagnostic test is perfect, and it is estimated that the use of this criterion with standard treadmill or bicycle ergometer stress testing produces (1) a rate of about 15% false-positive results in patients with apparently significant electrocardiographic changes during stress testing in whom angiography shows no significant coronary disease, and (2) about an equal number of false-negative results in patients with stress ECG changes that do not meet this criterion for significance but in whom angiography shows definite coronary artery disease.

Evaluating the slope of the ST segment improves matters somewhat (Plate 30). *Downsloping* ST segment depression is associated with a rate of only 5% to 10% false-positive results in middle-aged males undergoing stress testing and even less than that in those with a history of typical angina in whom chest pain occurs together with ST segment depression

Plate 31

Causes of ST Segment Depressions

Myocardial ischemia (see Plates 22 and 29)

Ventricular hypertrophy (see Plate 18)

Intraventricular conduction defects (see Plate 19)

Digitalis

Digitalis effect ⌐──────────────── Digitalis toxicity ──────────────┐

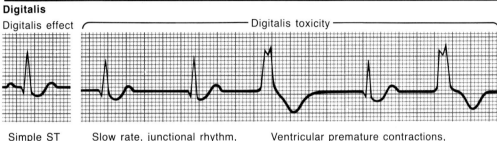

| Simple ST depression | Slow rate, junctional rhythm, other rhythm disturbances | Ventricular premature contractions, often bigeminal |

Other drugs

Nonspecific

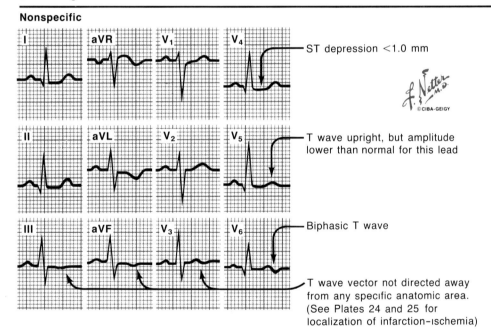

ST depression <1.0 mm

T wave upright, but amplitude lower than normal for this lead

Biphasic T wave

T wave vector not directed away from any specific anatomic area. (See Plates 24 and 25 for localization of infarction–ischemia)

during the stress test. *Horizontal* ST segment depression is also associated with a very low rate of false-positive results, while the error rate with *upsloping* ST segment depression is perhaps 30% to 40%, particularly in females, in persons without coronary risk factors, in those who do not have angina, and in those who do not have chest pain during the stress test.

Although ST segment depressions are often assumed to indicate ischemia, there are many other potential causes of this abnormality (Plate 31).

ST segment depressions, often associated with T wave inversions, are common with ventricular hypertrophy (usually in leads I, aVL, and V_4 through V_6 with left ventricular hypertrophy, and in leads V_1 and V_2 with right ventricular hypertrophy [Plate 18, Atlas ECGs 6-1 and 6-2]).

Both RBBB and LBBB are associated with major ST segment and T wave abnormalities, usually ST segment depressions and inverted T waves in the right precordial leads with RBBB and in leads I, aVL, and the left precordial leads with LBBB (Plate 19, Atlas ECGs 6-3 and 6-5).

A number of drugs affect the ECG. Patients with therapeutic blood levels of digitalis often have ST segment depressions, sometimes with flattening of T waves, which is termed "digitalis effect." These changes are usually not marked, often occur in many leads, and are present at rest as well as with exercise. However, the ST segment depression associated with digitalis can affect the results of an exercise stress test, and to eliminate any confusion, digitalis is generally stopped several days before diagnostic stress testing.

Digitalis toxicity has various effects on the ECG. In many patients, especially young persons with no ischemic heart disease, the primary manifestation of digitalis toxicity is likely to be bradyarrhythmia (sinus bradycardia with junctional rhythm) or various forms of AV block. Paroxysmal atrial tachycardia with $2:1$ AV block and VPCs are also common manifestations of digitalis toxicity. At times, VPCs may be bigeminal, and sometimes major ventricular arrhythmias occur. Many other drugs affect the ECG, particularly the ST segment and the T wave.

A very common electrocardiographic diagnosis is "nonspecific ST segment and T wave abnormalities," often abbreviated as "NS ST-T abn" (Plate 31, Atlas ECG 8-5). The term "nonspecific" implies that there is no known specific cause for the ST segment abnormalities; they are usually relatively minor and sometimes may be exceedingly subtle and subject to a good deal of interobserver variability. In order for ST-T abnormalities to be called "nonspecific," the ST depressions should be less than 1 mm, with generally upright T waves (that is, the T wave vector should be normal, since T wave vectors directed away from any specific anatomic area suggest ischemia in that area). (See Plates 24 and 25 for localization of myocardial ischemia.)

T Wave Abnormalities

The T wave in normal adults is upright in leads I, II and V_3 through V_6; inverted in lead aVR; and variable in leads III, aVL, aVF, V_1 and V_2. Table 2 gives the range of normal T wave amplitude.

Although T wave abnormalities often accompany abnormalities of the ST segment, in some instances only the T wave is affected (Plate 32). Abnormally tall and peaked T waves suggest either hyperkalemia or acute myocardial ischemia, for example, the earliest stages of acute myocardial infarction (Plate 32, top panel; Atlas ECGs 7-5, 7-8, and 8-6). Indeed, these two conditions may be pathophysiologically similar, since acute myocardial infarction is associated with cellular damage and potassium leakage from damaged cells, which probably causes localized hyperkalemia in the area of the infarction.

A high serum level of potassium causes many abnormalities in the ECG, including tall and peaked T waves and decreased P wave amplitude. At times, the P waves may be so small as to be invisible; the sinus node is still beating normally, but atrial depolarization has been so depressed by hyperkalemia that P waves are no longer seen.

The specialized atrial conduction tracts that conduct sinus impulses to the AV node are resistant to hyperkalemia, so that the SA node continues to

Plate 32

T Wave Abnormalities

Tall and peaked T waves

Hyperkalemia
  P wave often small or absent PR interval often prolonged QRS complex may be widened

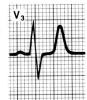

Acute myocardial ischemia
  Peaked T waves seen in earliest stages of acute infarction. ST segment elevation may be subtle, but usually becomes more obvious as infarction progresses

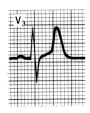

Flat T waves

Nonspecific etiology

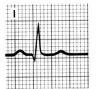 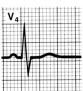

Inverted T waves

Myocardial ischemia (see Plate 29)
Subendocardial infarction (see Plate 23)
Myocardial disease
Chronic pericarditis (see Plate 27)
Ventricular hypertrophy (see Plate 18)
Intraventricular conduction defects (see Plate 19)
"Cerebral" T waves (e.g., subarachnoid hemorrhage)
Normal variant in some leads
Many other causes

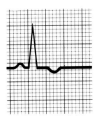

control the ventricles. Some electrocardiographers term this situation "sinoventricular rhythm." Hyperkalemia, then, is recognized by a rate characteristic of the SA node (60 to 100 beats per minute) rather than of the AV node or junction (40 to 55 beats per minute), with diminutive or absent P waves and with tall and peaked T waves. As hyperkalemia worsens, the PR interval may become prolonged and the QRS may be widened; the latter finding presages life-threatening hyperkalemia.

Flat T waves are seen in a number of situations and are usually termed "nonspecific" (Atlas ECG 8-7). Table 2 gives estimates for upper and lower limits of normal T wave amplitude in various leads.

Inverted T waves can be caused by a number of conditions, most notably myocardial ischemia and infarction (Atlas ECGs 7-7, 7-10, 7-12, and 8-8), but also including many cardiac (Atlas ECGs 6-1, 6-2, 6-3, 6-5, and 8-2) and noncardiac conditions. For example, significant cerebral disease such as subarachnoid hemorrhage may be associated with striking and widespread deeply inverted T waves; these are often termed "cerebral T waves" (Atlas ECG 8-9).

In some cases, T wave inversions are not pathologic at all. For example, in infants and children, T waves are normally inverted (sometimes strikingly so) in right precordial leads such as V_1, V_2 and V_3 (Atlas ECG 8-10). Although these T wave inversions usually disappear with advancing age (first in V_3, then in V_2, then in V_1), some adolescents and even young adults have a persistent pattern of right precordial T wave inversions. This

Table 2   T Wave Amplitude in Adults

Lead	Minimum (mm)	Maximum (mm)
I	−0.5	5.6
II	0	8.0
III	−2.0	5.5
aVR	−6.0	−1.0
aVL	−1.5	2.0
aVF	0.2	5.0
V_1	−3.0	5.0
V_2	2.0	12.0
V_3	2.0	16.0
V_4	1.6	14.0
V_5	1.0	10.0
V_6	1.0	6.0

is termed a "juvenile pattern" and is not associated with any cardiac pathology. It is generally unwise to make any etiologic cardiac diagnosis on the basis of T wave changes alone.

QT Interval Abnormalities

The QT interval is measured from the beginning of the QRS complex to the end of the T wave and varies with the heart rate. (For upper limits of normal for the QT interval, see chart, Plate 7.)

The QT interval may be prolonged by a number of conditions, including acute or chronic myocardial ischemia, myocarditis, antiarrhythmic agents (quinidine, procainamide, disopyramide, and others), psychotropic agents (phenothiazine, tricyclic antidepressants, and others), hypokalemia, hypomagnesemia, cerebral events such as subarachnoid hemorrhage, and other causes (Plate 33, Atlas ECG 8-11).

Excessively prolonged QT intervals are often associated with a dangerous form of ventricular tachycardia called "torsade de pointes," literally, "twisting of the points" (that is, twisting of the QRS axis). This arrhythmia shows periodic increasing and decreasing QRS amplitude, the result of the axis of the arrhythmia slowly turning around some imaginary point in the ventricle. Torsade de pointes, for all its elegant name and complicated pathophysiology, is not uncommon and often leads to cardiovascular collapse and death.

As noted, hypokalemia, hypomagnesemia, or hypocalcemia prolongs the QT interval. Hypocalcemia and hypomagnesemia primarily prolong the

---

Table 2 is adapted from Criteria Committee of the New York Heart Association. Nomenclature and Criteria for Diagnosis of Diseases of the Heart and Great Vessels. Eds. 6 and 8. Boston, Little Brown and Company, 1964 and 1979, based on Ferrer MI. Electrocardiographic Notebook. Ed 4. Mt. Kisco, NY, Futura Publishing Company, 1973, and on normal series studied by eight authors. Tables for normal P,Q,R, and S wave amplitudes, as well as for infants, children, and adolescents, are also given in these volumes.

Plate 33

QT Interval Abnormalities

Prolonged QT interval

Ischemia or acute or chronic myocardial disease

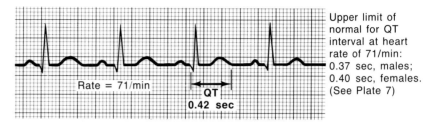

Rate = 71/min

QT
0.42 sec

Upper limit of normal for QT interval at heart rate of 71/min: 0.37 sec, males; 0.40 sec, females. (See Plate 7)

Drugs (quinidine, phenothiazines, others)

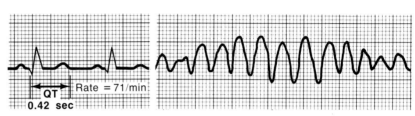

QT
0.42 sec
Rate = 71/min

QRS may be wide or of low amplitude. T wave may be flat

May progress to torsade de pointes or other serious arrhythmia

Hypocalcemia (or hypomagnesemia)

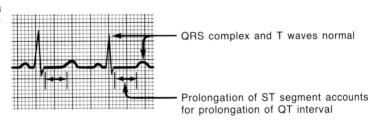

QRS complex and T waves normal

Prolongation of ST segment accounts for prolongation of QT interval

Hypokalemia

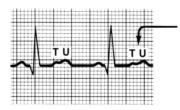

T U   T U

Low T wave merges with high U wave to create apparent prolongation of QT interval

Shortened QT interval

Hypercalcemia

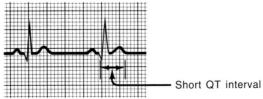

Short QT interval

ST segment, whereas hypokalemia causes low-amplitude T waves and unusually large U waves, which merge to create a single T-U wave and apparent QT interval prolongation. Finally, some persons may have congenital prolongation of the QT interval, which is associated with major ventricular arrhythmias and sudden cardiac death.

Although the physician should refer to a chart for the upper limits of normal of QT intervals of any given heart rate, a good rule of thumb is that QT intervals >0.40 second in males and >0.44 second in females are abnormal when heart rate exceeds 60/minute, and QT intervals >0.60 second are the likely cause of major ventricular arrhythmia in a patient with such extreme QT prolongation. The QT interval is shortened in hypercalcemia and in the presence of very rapid heart rates (Atlas ECG 8-12).

9 BASIC PACEMAKER ELECTROCARDIOGRAPHY

Rapid and continuing advances in the field of cardiac pacing have made a basic understanding of new pacemakers a requirement for those involved in the interpretation of ECGs. The first step in acquiring this knowledge is learning the Inter-Society Commission for Heart Disease (ICHD) pacemaker identification code, which succinctly describes pacing *modes*. Although the ICHD code has five positions, it is most commonly used in the abbreviated three-position form shown in Table 3.

Each letter in the three-position ICHD code refers to a specific function of the pacemaker. The combined three-letter identification code results in the specification of a particular pacing mode.

Position I refers to the chamber(s) *paced*. Single-chamber pacemakers may pace either the ventricle (V) or the atrium (A), while dual-chamber pacemakers may pace both chambers, receiving a dual (D) designation.

Position II refers to the chamber(s) *sensed* by the pacemaker's sensing amplifiers. These amplifiers detect spontaneous *intrinsic* depolarizations in the heart, namely, P waves in the atrium or QRS complexes in the ventricle. Single-chamber pacemakers may sense either in the atrium (A) or in the ventricle (V), while certain (but not all) dual-chamber pacemakers sense in both chambers, receiving a dual (D) designation.

Table 3   Inter-Society Commission for Heart Disease (ICHD) Code

Position Designation	I Chamber paced	II Chamber sensed	III Response to sensing
Letters used	**V**—ventricle	**V**—ventricle	**I**—inhibited
	A—atrium	**A**—atrium	**T**—triggered
	D—dual	**D**—dual	**D**—dual*
	O—none	**O**—none	**O**—none

*Atrial triggered and atrial/ventricular inhibited

The "O" designation in position II means that the pacemaker's sensing amplifiers have been turned off and that the device will pace at the programmed rate regardless of the heart's intrinsic rhythm. By convention, when the O is placed in position II, position III is assigned the O designation as well.

Position III refers to the pacemaker's *response* to a sensed P wave or QRS complex. Most single-chamber pacemakers respond to a sensed P wave or QRS by *inhibiting (I)*. That is, the pacemaker timer is reset, and no pacemaker stimulus is delivered to the heart for a preprogrammed interval. The *triggered (T)* mode is seldom used in single-chamber pacemakers except for testing or other special situations. Triggering results in the delivery of a pacemaker stimulus in response to a sensed P wave or QRS.

Dual-chamber pacemakers may use both triggering *and* inhibition, and therefore receive the dual (D) designation. These pacemakers trigger the ventricular stimulus just after spontaneous P waves, producing synchrony between the chambers. AV universal (DDD) pacemakers also *inhibit* in the atrium and ventricle when spontaneous complexes are sensed. This prevents competition between paced and spontaneous rhythms.

VVI (Ventricular Demand or Ventricular Inhibited) Pacing

Plate 34A is a schematic diagram showing the essential components of a VVI pacing system. The pacing lead is inserted in the right ventricle and connects to the pacemaker generator. The pacemaker generator itself has two components, a pacing amplifier and a sensing amplifier. A VVI pacemaker *paces* in the ventricle (ICHD code position I = V), *senses* in the ventricle (position II = V), and *inhibits* in response to a sensed QRS (position III = I).

Plate 34B shows typical VVI pacemaker function. The pacemaker amplifier is programmed to pace at a particular rate with a particular *automatic* interval between impulses. When the sensing amplifier detects an intrinsic QRS complex (a VPC in this example), it inhibits the pacing amplifier, which resumes pacing after the escape interval. Usually, the automatic and *escape* intervals are of equal duration.

Plate 34C shows the response of the VVI pacemaker to an increase in the patient's sinus rate with activity. While the patient is at rest with a sinus rate lower than the pacemaker's preset rate, the pacemaker maintains its programmed rate, which also is known as the *lower rate limit*. However, as the sinus rate increases, the VVI pacemaker does not follow. This is immaterial in a patient with normal AV conduction, but in a patient with complete heart block, the ventricular rate cannot rise normally (Plate 35D). Thus, VVI is *not* a rate-responsive pacing mode.

Plate 35E shows what happens when a strong magnet of the type supplied with pacemakers is applied over the site of the pacemaker. A magnetic reed switch is closed inside the pacemaker, which turns off the sensing amplifier. In ICHD terminology, the device goes into the VOO mode. In VOO, the patient's intrinsic QRS complexes are not sensed, and pacemaker spikes are delivered asynchronously. Whenever the pacing stimulus falls at a time when the ventricular myocardium is nonrefractory, a paced QRS complex results. The magnetic rate (which is not always the same as the

Plate 34

Single–Chamber Ventricular Pacing

A. VVI (ventricular demand or ventricular inhibited) pacing

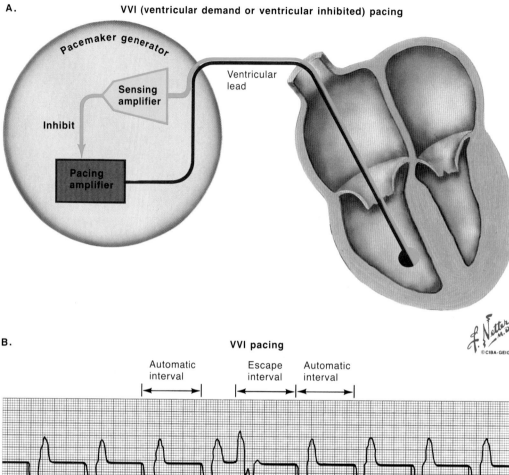

B. VVI pacing

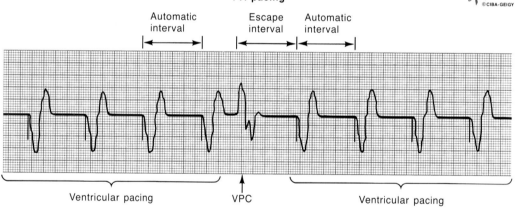

Automatic interval | Escape interval | Automatic interval

Ventricular pacing   VPC   Ventricular pacing

C. VVI pacing with increasing atrial rate and normal AV conduction

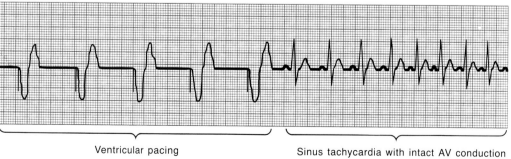

Ventricular pacing   Sinus tachycardia with intact AV conduction

Plate 35

Single-Chamber Ventricular Pacing (continued)

D.   **VVI pacing with increasing atrial rate and complete heart block**

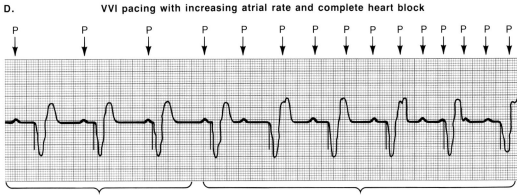

Ventricular pacing: atrial rate slower than lower rate limit of pacemaker

Ventricular pacing at same (slow) rate: atrial rate faster than lower rate limit of pacemaker, but complete heart block prevents atrial activity from influencing ventricles or pacemaker

E.   **VOO pacing with pacemaker magnet application over VVI pacemaker**

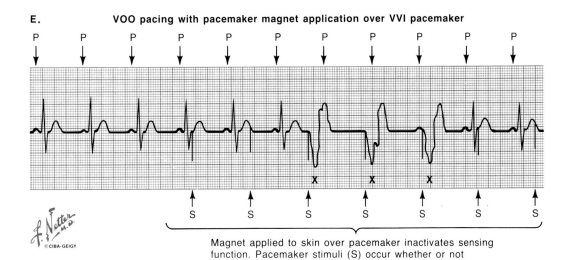

Magnet applied to skin over pacemaker inactivates sensing function. Pacemaker stimuli (S) occur whether or not intrinsic beats are present, but capture (pace) ventricle only when ventricle is not refractory from an intrinsic beat (X = pacemaker capture beats, P = intrinsic atrial P waves)

paced rate) is often used as an index of the pacemaker battery's condition. A slowing of the magnetic rate from specification indicates impending battery depletion and a need for elective generator replacement.

Application of a magnet allows confirmation that the pacemaker is actually capable of pacing when it has been continuously inhibited by the patient's intrinsic rhythm. Conversely, the intrinsic complexes in a patient who is continuously paced may be exposed when a magnet is applied.

DVI (AV Sequential) Pacing

Plate 36A is a schematic representation of a DVI pacemaker. With DVI pacing, pacemaker leads are connected to both the atrium and ventricle; thus, the term "dual-chamber pacing" applies. Both the atrium and the ventricle may be paced (position I = D), while only the ventricle is attached to a sensing amplifier (position II = V). When an intrinsic QRS complex is detected by the ventricular sensing amplifier, both the atrial and ventricular pacing amplifiers are inhibited (position III = I). This pacemaker is there-fore "blind" to atrial activity, and competition between atrial intrinsic and atrial paced beats may occur.

Plate 36B shows an example of a DVI pacemaker beginning to pace at its rate of 60 as the sinus rhythm slows. This is a *noncommitted* DVI pace-maker, in that the pacemaker is not "committed" to a ventricular stimulus after an atrial stimulus has been emitted. Thus, as long as the intrinsic PR interval is shorter than the pacemaker's programmed AV interval, conduc-tion proceeds normally through the AV node (beats 3 to 6), and intrinsic conducted ventricular beats inhibit the ventricular pacemaker. As AV con-duction slows and the intrinsic PR interval exceeds the pacemaker's pro-grammed PR interval, both atria and ventricles are paced (beats 7 to 10).

Some DVI pacemakers are *committed*; that is, they must deliver a ven-tricular stimulus once an atrial stimulus has been delivered. This is one technique used to prevent abnormal ventricular inhibition of the pacemaker due to *crosstalk* from the atrial pacemaker stimulus. (Crosstalk occurs when the ventricular sensing amplifier detects the atrial pacing stimulus and mis-interprets it as an intrinsic ventricular QRS.)

Plate 36C illustrates two important negative features of DVI pacing. First, in this example of complete heart block, the fact that the DVI pacemaker is "blind" to intrinsic atrial activity is evident. As the sinus P wave rate increases, beats 4 through 9 show competitive atrial paced stimuli occur-ring shortly after intrinsic atrial beats. Such atrial competition may in some cases increase the likelihood of atrial fibrillation.

Second, despite the fact that the sinus P wave rate has increased, it is apparent that the ventricular paced rate remains constant at the pace-maker's programmed rate (lower rate limit). Thus, like VVI, DVI is *not* a rate-responsive pacing mode.

DDD (AV Universal) Pacing

Plate 37A is a schematic representation of a DDD pacemaker. As the ICHD code indicates, both the atria and the ventricles are paced (position I = D), and both atria and ventricles are sensed (position II = D). Sensing may result in inhibition or triggering (position III = D); VPCs inhibit ventricular pacing, while P waves trigger a ventricular stimulus after a programmed AV interval.

Plate 37B shows the operation of a DDD pacemaker over a range of atrial rates. When the intrinsic atrial rate tries to fall below the programmed *lower rate limit*, the atrial pacemaker channel begins to pace at the lower rate limit. If, as in this example, the pacemaker's programmed AV interval is shorter than the intrinsic conduction time down the heart's AV node, the ventricular pacemaker channel also paces the ventricle (beats 1 and 2). Thus, the DDD pacemaker behaves like a DVI pacemaker when the intrin-sic atrial rate tends to be slower than the pacemaker's lower rate limit.

When the intrinsic atrial rate begins to rise above the lower rate limit, as in physical exercise, the atrial channel is inhibited and the ventricular pac-ing channel begins to track the intrinsic atrial rate. This represents *atrial*

Plate 36

Dual–Chamber Pacing

A.

DVI (AV sequential) pacing

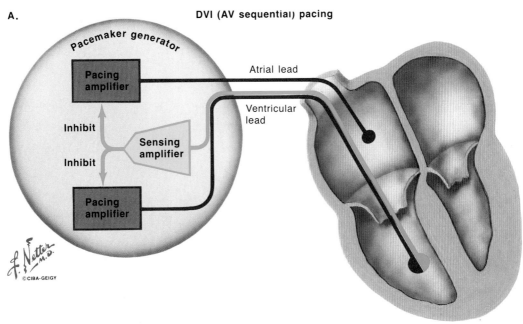

Pacemaker generator

Pacing amplifier

Atrial lead

Ventricular lead

Inhibit

Sensing amplifier

Inhibit

Pacing amplifier

B.

Noncommitted DVI pacing

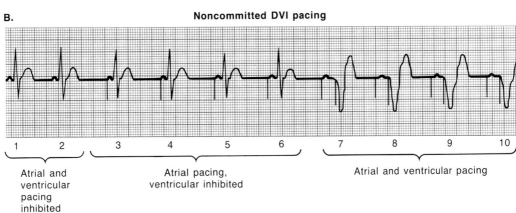

1 2 3 4 5 6 7 8 9 10

Atrial and ventricular pacing inhibited

Atrial pacing, ventricular inhibited

Atrial and ventricular pacing

C.

DVI pacing with competition between intrinsic and paced atrial (P) waves

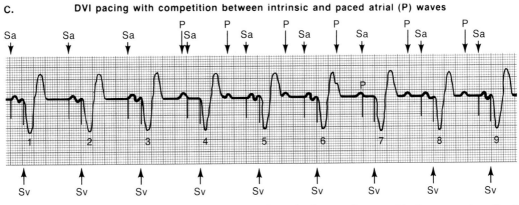

Sa   Sa   Sa   P Sa   P Sa   P Sa   P Sa   P Sa   P Sa

1 2 3 4 5 6 7 8 9

Sv   Sv   Sv   Sv   Sv   Sv   Sv   Sv   Sv

P = intrinsic atrial P waves   Sa = atrial pacemaker stimuli   Sv = ventricular pacemaker stimuli

Plate 37

Dual-Chamber Pacing (continued)

A.   DDD (AV universal) pacing

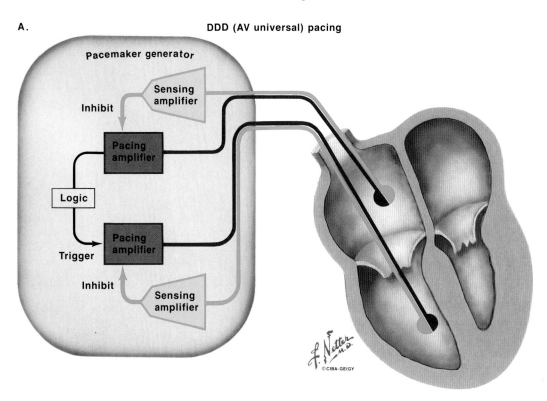

B.   DDD pacing

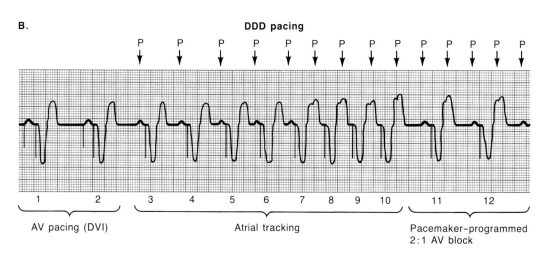

(P = intrinsic atrial P wave)

tracking, or *rate responsiveness* (beats 3 to 10). In contrast to the other pacemakers already discussed, the DDD pacemaker allows a patient with complete heart block to raise his ventricular rate with activity.

The DDD pacemaker tracks an atrial rate only up to a certain maximum, known as the *upper rate limit*. Beyond the upper rate limit, pacemakers can exhibit variable degrees of simulated second-degree block or declines in

Plate 38

Complication of Dual–Chamber Pacing

Endless loop tachycardia with DDD pacemaker

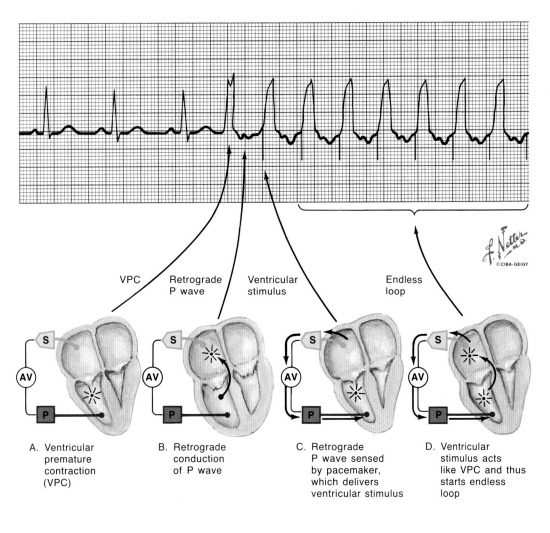

VPC Retrograde P wave Ventricular stimulus Endless loop

A. Ventricular premature contraction (VPC)

B. Retrograde conduction of P wave

C. Retrograde P wave sensed by pacemaker, which delivers ventricular stimulus

D. Ventricular stimulus acts like VPC and thus starts endless loop

S = atrial sensing amplifier   **AV** = pacemaker AV delay   **P** = ventricular pacing amplifier

ventricular paced rate according to predetermined logic. The parameters that determine the upper rate response can be programmed into the pacemaker (in this example, 2:1 AV block is programmed when P wave rate exceeds 140/minute — beats 11 to 12).

Plate 38 demonstrates one of the common complications of DDD pacing, *pacemaker-mediated endless loop tachycardia* (PM-ELT). A DDD pacemaker contains the necessary electrical components to simulate an accessory bypass tract around the AV node. That is, the pacemaker senses atrial activity and then stimulates the ventricle along an electrical pathway independent of the AV node. Thus, the pacemaker represents the equivalent of an implanted WPW syndrome (page 27).

Table 4 Features of Commonly Used Pacemakers

Common name	ICHD code	Chamber paced	Chamber sensed	Response to sensing	Advantages	Disadvantages
Ventricular demand pacemaker	VVI	Ventricle	Ventricle	Inhibits (pacer shuts off if intrinsic ventricular beat occurs)	Simplest Cheapest Single ventricular beat only Little chance of competitive rhythms	Not rate-responsive Loss of synchronized AV conduction and atrial "kick" may reduce cardiac output
AV sequential pacemaker	DVI	Atrium and ventricle	Ventricle	Same as VVI	Synchronized AV conduction with atrial "kick" optimizes cardiac output	Requires atrial and ventricular leads Not rate-responsive Since "blind" to intrinsic atrial activity (no atrial sensing), competitive atrial rhythms and even atrial fibrillation may occur
AV universal pacemaker	DDD	Atrium and ventricle	Atrium and ventricle	Paces ventricle in response to atrial sensed complex; inhibits ventricle in response to ventricular sensed complex	Synchronized AV conduction and rate-responsive	Most expensive Requires atrial and ventricular leads Possibility of endless loop tachycardia

The basis for PM-ELT is the ability of the AV node to conduct retrograde from the ventricle up to the atrium. Two-thirds of patients with sick sinus syndrome can do this, and even one-third of patients with antegrade complete heart block are capable of retrograde conduction.

In Plate 38, a VPC (A) conducts retrograde up the AV node and produces a retrograde P wave (B). This P wave is sensed by the pacemaker atrial sensing amplifier, and after the programmed AV interval, the ventricle is paced (C). The paced ventricular complex now conducts back up the AV node and produces another retrograde P wave, completing the loop (D). This endless loop repeats over and over, producing the PM-ELT until the AV node fatigues or some other intervention is made.

PM-ELT will not start as long as the atrium and ventricle beat in synchrony with a normal AV interval, because the AV node is normally refractory in the retrograde direction when it has recently been depolarized. The example shown is PM-ELT produced by a VPC, but any event that produces dissociation between the atrium and the ventricle may allow the AV node to recover from refractoriness and permit PM-ELT.

Modern DDD pacemakers have several features that can help prevent PM-ELT. The most effective is the programmable atrial refractory period of the atrial sensing amplifier. During the pacemaker's atrial refractory period, the atrial sensing amplifier is "turned off" and does not sense any P waves. As long as the atrial refractory period (as measured from the last ventricular complex) is longer than the retrograde AV conduction time, the retrograde P wave is not sensed, and PM-ELT cannot be initiated.

The maximum atrial tracking rate of a DDD pacemaker is determined by the sum of the AV interval (AVI) and the atrial refractory period (ARP), because any P wave that comes within these periods is not sensed by the pacemaker and does not trigger a ventricular stimulus. Thus, increasing protection against retrograde P waves by lengthening the atrial refractory period reduces the upper rate limit of the pacemaker. In Plate 37B, the upper rate response is the abrupt development of 2:1 AV block. Certain pacemakers allow separate programming of an upper rate limit to a rate below the maximum set by the sum of AVI + ARP. Table 4 summarizes features of commonly used pacemakers.

This atlas includes actual ECGs that illustrate points made in the preceding sections. Unless otherwise specified, all ECGs are reproduced in the format of Figure 1.

Modern electrocardiographs generally provide an automatic standardization pulse in the shape of a square wave, verifying that 1 mv produces exactly 10-mm upward deflection (three solid arrows at right in Figure 1). If an older electrocardiograph is used, the operator should always adjust the standardization before taking the ECG and record the standardization pulse at the beginning of the tracing.

The electrocardiographs currently in use usually inscribe four groups of three leads. From left to right, the lead groups are I, II, III; aVR, aVL, aVF; V_1, V_2, V_3; and V_4, V_5, V_6. The three leads in each group are recorded simultaneously, and the entire tracing is usually continuous; that is, notwithstanding the lead switching that occurs automatically between groups of three leads, the entire tracing can be used for analysis of rate or rhythm. For example, the RR interval measured between the last complex in lead I and the first complex in lead aVR is accurate in spite of the intervening lead switch: the electrocardiograph records continuously in real time and switches essentially instantaneously from the first set of leads to the subsequent set. Some electrocardiographs produce artifacts at the moment of lead switches (broken arrows in Figure 1). Such artifacts should not be confused with QRS complexes, pacemaker spikes, or other true electrocardiographic deflections.

FIGURE 1

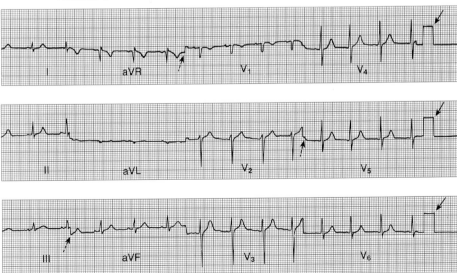

All ECGs in this section are 50% of actual size.

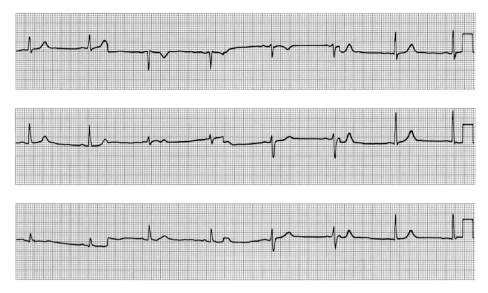

ECG 5-1. Sinus bradycardia, rate 45. Although rate limits for normal sinus rhythm are traditionally given as 60 to 100/minute, sinus rates below 60 are frequently normal. Physical conditioning, for example, increases stroke volume and usually decreases resting heart rate. Many normal athletes have low resting heart rates, often sinus bradycardia with rates in the 50s and even 40s. This ECG was recorded in a healthy 23-year-old, and is a normal variant.

ECG 5-2. Sinus tachycardia, rate 119.

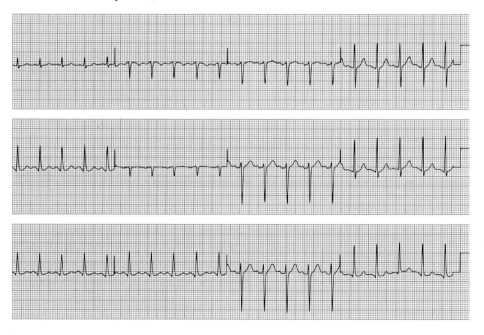

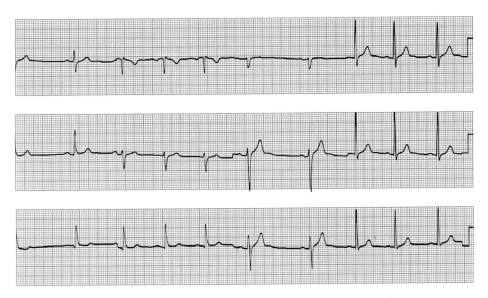

ECG 5-3. Sinus arrhythmia, or sinus irregularity. Despite the fact that PP intervals vary by ≥0.16 second, all P waves and PR intervals are identical in any single lead. This is important in differentiating sinus irregularity (a normal variant) from wandering atrial pacemaker or multifocal atrial tachycardia.

ECG 5-4. Nonsinus atrial (coronary sinus) rhythm. P wave axis is highly unusual, directed superiorly and leftward, that is, from the direction of the AV node backward toward the SA node. Note the inverted P waves in leads II, III and aVF. The PR interval and heart rate are normal.

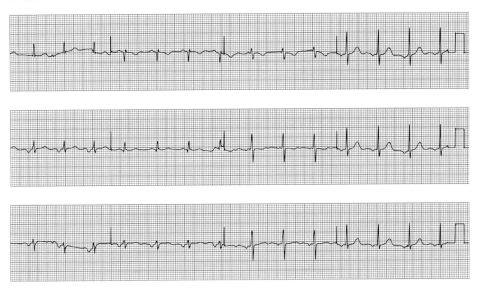

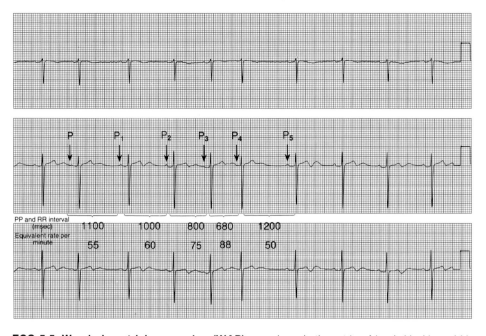

PP and RR interval (msec)	1100	1000	800	680	1200
Equivalent rate per minute	55	60	75	88	50

ECG 5-5. Wandering atrial pacemaker (WAP) seen in a rhythm strip of leads V_1, V_2 and V_3 only. Atrial depolarization originates not from a single location such as the sinus node, but from many different locations. Thus, P waves have at least five separate shapes (P_1, P_2, P_3, P_4, P_5). Since depolarization originates in differing locations, spread throughout the atrium follows differing pathways (thus, variable shapes of P waves) and requires variable amounts of time to completely penetrate the atrium and reach the AV node (thus, variable PR intervals). The various atrial sites may have different rates of depolarization, and thus PP (and therefore RR) rates also vary. ($PP_1 = 1100$ msec, equivalent to a rate of 55/minute. P_1P_2 is equivalent to a rate of 60, P_2P_3 to 75, P_3P_4 to 88, and P_4P_5 to 50.) This irregularly irregular rhythm might be mistaken for atrial fibrillation unless careful study identifies the several different P waves. At least three different P wave morphologies are required for the diagnosis of WAP; otherwise, the rhythm might simply be sinus rhythm with atrial premature contractions.

ECG 5-6. Multifocal atrial tachycardia (MAT). As with wandering atrial pacemaker, several different P wave shapes (P_1, P_2, P_3, P_4), PR intervals, and PP/RR intervals are seen. The differentiation between WAP and MAT is not entirely clear but often is made arbitrarily on the basis of rate: WAP if ventricular rate is <100/minute; MAT if >100/minute.

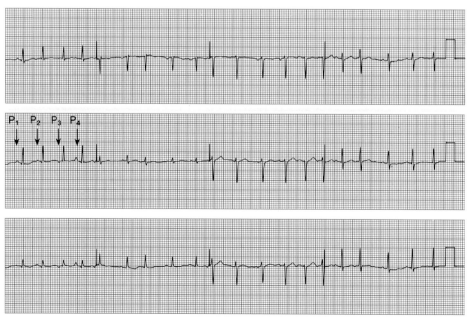

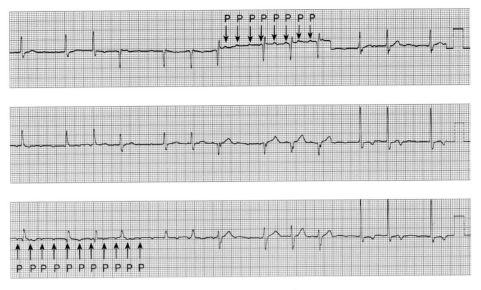

ECG 5-7. Paroxysmal atrial tachycardia (PAT) with variable AV block. With fewer QRS complexes because of the AV block, the rapid P waves are easily seen (arrows). Note that AV block in this situation is not necessarily pathologic but is often physiologic in protecting the ventricle from overly rapid atrial rates. In this tracing, the atrial rate is 215/minute, which would be exceedingly dangerous if 1:1 AV conduction were present, but the AV block results in a ventricular rate of 63.

ECG 5-8. Paroxysmal atrial tachycardia with 1:1 AV conduction, or supraventricular tachycardia. With 1:1 conduction, P waves usually fall on the preceding T wave and may be extremely difficult to identify. This type of tracing — a very rapid tachycardia with narrow QRS complexes and no definite P waves — is often called supraventricular tachycardia, which indicates that the exact site of origin of rhythm is uncertain, although clearly above the ventricle since the QRS complexes are narrow. This tracing is probably PAT, given its rate of 168; however, it could be junctional or sinus tachycardia (the rate would be unusually fast for either) or conceivably atrial flutter with 2:1 AV block (except that flutter waves, "F" waves, are frequently not difficult to identify, particularly in lead III, aVF or V_1). Unless antiarrhythmic drugs have been given, F waves are so characteristically at or near a rate of 300 that with 2:1 AV block, the QRS rate is usually very close to 150, rather slower than the rate here or in most instances of PAT.

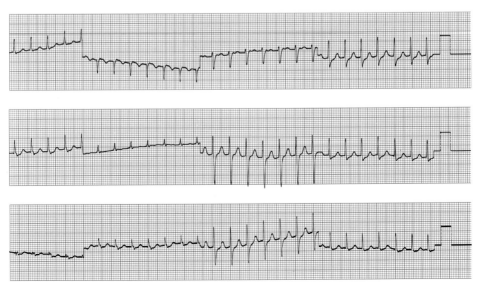

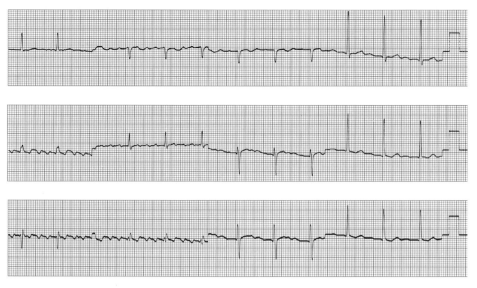

ECG 5-9. Atrial flutter with 4:1 AV block. Continuously undulating F waves with no isoelectric baseline are best seen in leads II, III and aVF. Although the contour of all F waves is identical, some are deformed by falling on a QRS or T wave, and thus may seem to have a different appearance. The atrial rate is 300, and the ventricular rate is 75.

ECG 5-10. Atrial flutter-fibrillation. In some areas (solid arrows), this rhythm resembles atrial flutter, with reasonably high-amplitude atrial depolarizations that resemble F waves. However, in other areas, the atrial activity is much less organized (broken arrow). The ventricular response, irregularly irregular, is much more characteristic of atrial fibrillation than atrial flutter. Although the differentiation between flutter and flutter-fibrillation is not terribly important, true atrial flutter tends to be quite sensitive to electroshock and frequently can be converted to sinus rhythm with very low-energy shock. Flutter-fibrillation behaves like atrial fibrillation and requires much higher energy levels for cardioversion.

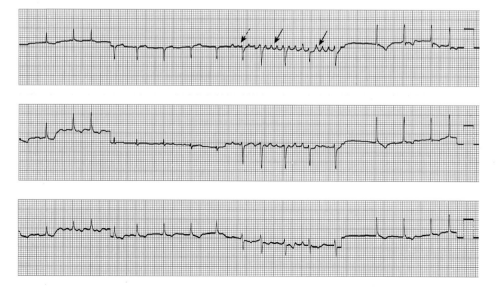

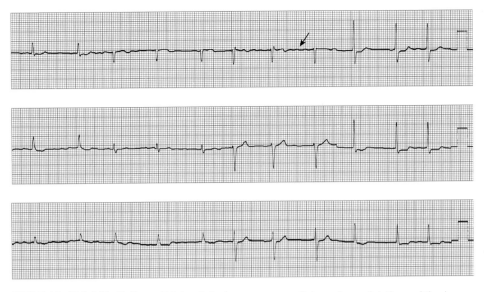

ECG 5-11. Atrial fibrillation. Atrial activity is seen as small, irregular undulations of the baseline in lead V$_1$ (arrow). Often, the atrial activity in atrial fibrillation may be impossible to identify on a standard ECG. In either case, the absence of obvious P waves and the irregularly irregular response of QRS complexes generally make the diagnosis obvious.

ECG 5-12. "Mid" junctional rhythm, often simply "junctional rhythm" without qualification. No P waves are visible because they are buried in the middle of QRS complexes. (This could be proved with a His bundle intracardiac tracing.) Absence of P waves; a rate between 40 and 55 (43 in this tracing); and regular, reasonably narrow QRS complexes make the diagnosis of junctional rhythm likely. (Actually, the QRS is somewhat wide, and an intraventricular block is also present here.) Fine atrial fibrillation may also produce an ECG in which no atrial activity is discernible (that is, no P waves can be identified), but irregularity of QRS complexes differentiates atrial fibrillation from junctional rhythm.

Caution should be exercised if the ventricular response of atrial fibrillation is slow, since small but definite irregularities may not be apparent to the eye and measurement of several RR intervals may be needed to determine whether ventricular response is regular (junctional rhythm) or irregular (atrial fibrillation).

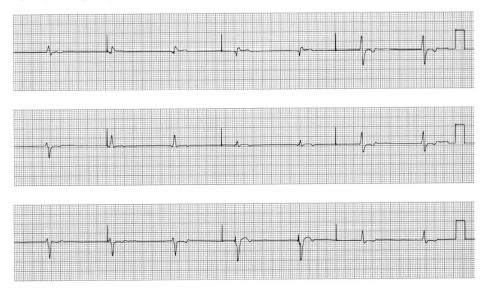

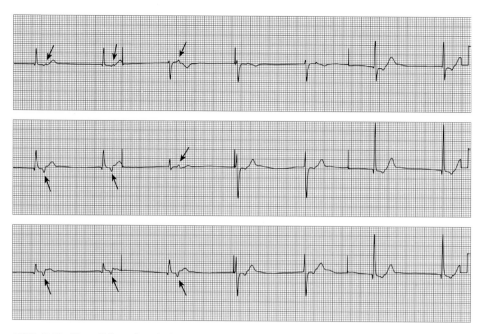

ECG 5-13. "Low" junctional rhythm. The site of initial depolarization is located within the AV node, close enough to the ventricle so that the ventricle is depolarized first, and then atrial depolarization follows. Thus, the P waves (arrows) follow the QRS complexes. When junctional rhythm is referred to, "high," "mid," and "low" are cited in quotation marks, since the actual anatomic location of initial depolarization may not always be "high," "mid," or "low" in the AV node. Both the electrophysiologic location and the relative time required for depolarization to travel up to the atrium or down to the ventricle determine whether the P waves precede, are buried in, or follow the QRS complexes. The rate of this ECG is slow, 40/minute, typical of the intrinsic rate of the junction.

ECG 5-14. Junctional tachycardia. As in junctional rhythm, P waves are hidden in QRS complexes, but QRS complexes are narrow and perfectly regular. The rate (118 here) is considerably above the intrinsic rate of the AV node or junction (40 to 55/minute), so that this is junctional tachycardia.

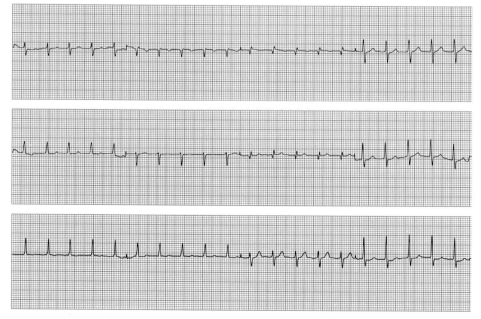

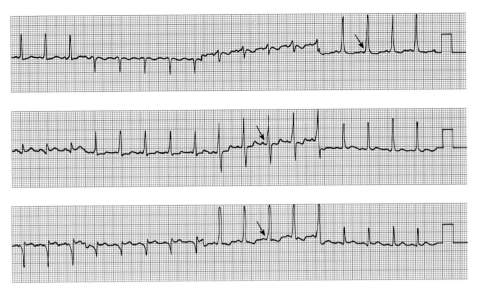

ECG 5-15. Normal sinus rhythm with Wolff-Parkinson-White (WPW) syndrome type A.
The QRS is wide (0.14 second). However, the WPW syndrome has several additional important characteristics: short PR interval (0.11 second) and the slurred upstroke at the beginning of the QRS complex called the delta wave, best seen in leads V_2, V_3 and V_4 (arrows).

In this patient, the abnormal bypass tract is located posteriorly, which means that the abnormal early depolarization of a small portion of the ventricle via the bypass tract, rather than by the usual AV node-His-Purkinje ventricular conduction system, occurs anteriorly. Thus, if one calculates the axis of the abnormal early portion of the QRS complex (the delta wave or wave of "preexcitation"), it would be directed anteriorly, toward the right precordial leads. This ECG demonstrates a prominent upward sloping delta wave in leads V_1 through V_4. Although large Q waves are seen in leads II, III and aVF, these are the result of the abnormal conduction pathway and do not represent inferior myocardial infarction.

ECG 5-16. Normal sinus rhythm with Wolff-Parkinson-White syndrome type B. In WPW type B, the abnormal bypass tract is located anteriorly, giving a delta wave at the beginning of the QRS complex directed posteriorly, or generally toward leads V_5 and V_6. Again note the wide QRS (0.14 second), short PR interval (0.11 second), and delta waves (negative delta wave in the anteriorly placed lead V_1 and positive delta waves in the posteriorly placed leads V_5 and V_6 [arrows]).

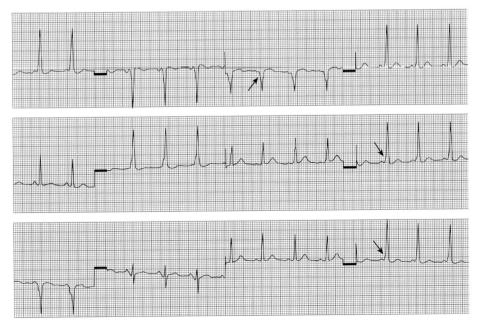

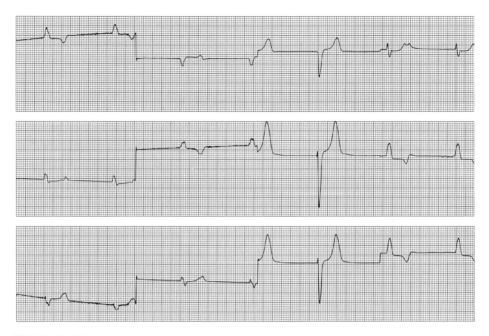

ECG 5-17. Idioventricular rhythm. The QRS is very wide (0.15 second); there are no P waves, and the rate is 39, within the usual range of idioventricular pacemakers (20 to 40/minute). There are also ST depressions and T wave inversions in leads I, aVL, V_5 and V_6, probably related to the abnormal pattern of impulse generation and conduction. At times, ST-T abnormalities may be so marked as to appear bizarre. This is frequently a dangerous, unstable, and at times preterminal rhythm, as its emergence implies that all higher pacemakers (SA node, atrium, AV node) are not functioning. With extremely slow ventricular rates and lack of atrial activity, serious hemodynamic derangements, including hypotension, shock, and circulatory collapse, are not uncommon.

ECG 5-18. Accelerated idioventricular rhythm (AIVR) from a 24-hour ambulatory ECG recording. Again, the QRS is wide, and there are no P waves, suggesting a ventricular origin of this rhythm. However, the rate is faster than the usual intrinsic rate of an idioventricular pacemaker. Adverse hemodynamic consequences are unusual; indeed, patients are often unaware of AIVR. It usually occurs in short bursts, often 4 to 20 consecutive beats, and is quite common in the first few days after acute myocardial infarction.

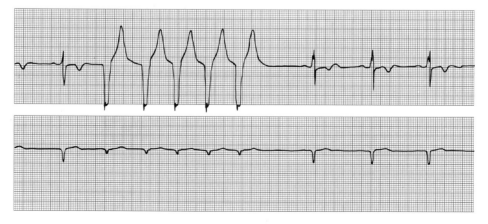

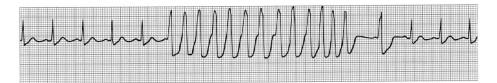

ECG 5-19. Normal sinus rhythm with a burst of ventricular tachycardia from a coronary care unit monitor strip. ECG shows wide, bizarre QRS complexes, with T waves usually opposite in direction to the major QRS deflection; rate is about 180/minute. There are often slight irregularities in the rate of ventricular tachycardia and, not infrequently, a gradual acceleration from the first few beats to subsequent beats. Short bursts of ventricular tachycardia may or may not be perceived by the patient or have hemodynamic consequences; readers of 24-hour ambulatory ECGs frequently see short asymptomatic bursts of ventricular tachycardia. Whether or not short runs of ventricular tachycardia are dangerous is a complicated evaluation related to ventricular function; the presence or absence of active ischemic heart disease, particularly recent acute myocardial infarction; and various other factors.

ECG 5-20. Sustained ventricular tachycardia and ventricular fibrillation in a continuous rhythm strip. Wide QRS complexes with no discernible P waves at a rate of 312/minute begin after a ventricular premature contraction (VPC) falls on the T wave (R on T VPC) of the sixth beat of supraventricular tachycardia at top left. Sustained ventricular tachycardia generally causes symptoms, sometimes no more than an awareness of palpitations, but often including extreme weakness, dizziness, syncope, or even circulatory collapse. In the middle of the center strip, ventricular tachycardia degenerates into ventricular fibrillation (VF). Ventricular fibrillation has no organized QRS complexes, even though, as in this example of very recent-onset ventricular fibrillation, undulations of the baseline may be visible. It is, of course, the rhythm usually associated with cardiac arrest and leads to death within a few minutes.

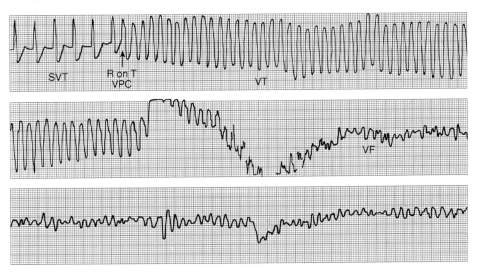

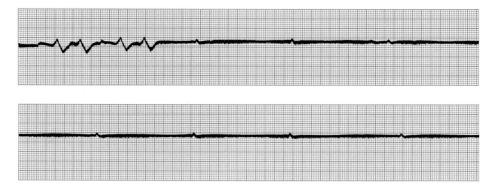

ECG 5-21. Ventricular standstill in a continuous rhythm strip. P waves and four wide, bizarre QRS complexes are seen at top left. Then, in the center of the top rhythm strip, P waves continue but there is no ventricular activity whatever. The baseline, aside from the P waves and some 60-cycle electrical interference, is perfectly flat, without the fine or coarse undulations often seen in ventricular fibrillation. Ventricular standstill, of course, also causes cardiac arrest and rapid death.

In many ways, standstill is even more ominous than ventricular fibrillation, since the latter is sometimes a random electrical event that if treated with immediate defibrillation, is compatible with survival and with subsequent good ventricular function. Standstill, on the other hand, implies inability of all potential pacemakers within the heart to depolarize. This is generally associated with massive myocardial damage, sometimes the end result of many minutes of untreated ventricular fibrillation, with consequent widespread myocardial cell death.

ECG 5-22. Normal sinus rhythm with first-degree AV block. The PR interval is constant at 0.32 second. Every P wave is associated with a conducted QRS complex.

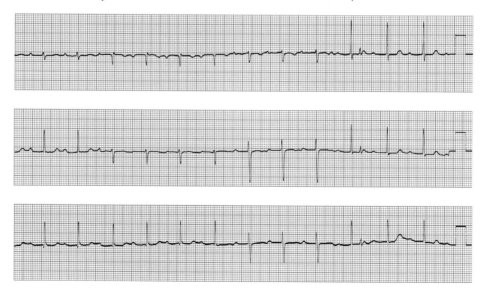

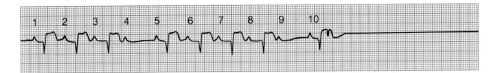

ECG 5-23. Second-degree AV block: Mobitz type I (Wenckebach), progressive lengthening of the PR interval until conduction fails and a QRS is dropped. The PR interval is 0.24 second in beat 1, 0.29 second in beat 2, and 0.35 second in beat 3; then, the fourth P wave fails to conduct. Given time for the AV node to recover, the following beat 5 has a shorter PR interval of 0.25 second, which again increases progressively until another beat is dropped at 9. Since some P waves conduct while some do not, this is incomplete, or second-degree, heart block. In left hand group of beats, there are four P waves for three QRS complexes; at right, there are five P waves for four QRS complexes, often written as 4:3 and 5:4 Wenckebach, respectively. The anatomic site of the Wenckebach type of second-degree heart block is generally at the crest of the AV node. Should this progress to complete heart block, a junctional escape rhythm with narrow QRS complexes and an adequate ventricular rate would be expected.

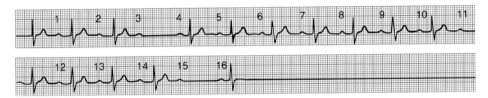

ECG 5-24. Second-degree AV block: Mobitz type II (non-Wenckebach). The PR interval is reasonably constant at 0.29 second throughout most of this continuous rhythm strip; beats are suddenly dropped at 3 and 15 (although the PR interval increases somewhat in the beat just preceding and decreases somewhat in the beat immediately following the dropped beats). Again, since some P waves conduct to the ventricle and some do not, this is incomplete, or second-degree, heart block. The anatomic site of Mobitz II heart block is probably in the His bundle or the Purkinje system; thus, if this type of incomplete heart block becomes complete heart block, the AV node is cut off from the ventricles and the escape rhythm will be ventricular with wide QRS complexes and a slow, often inadequate idioventricular rate. Mobitz II heart block is thus considerably more dangerous than Mobitz I (Wenckebach) incomplete (second-degree) heart block.

ECG 5-25. 2:1 AV block. In the situation in which every other P wave is blocked, it is impossible to tell whether or not the PR interval is progressively increasing (since there is never more than one completed PR interval at a time). Thus, one cannot differentiate between Mobitz I and Mobitz II, and it is unclear whether the site of block is at the crest of the AV node or in the His-Purkinje system. If this differentiation is clinically vital, intracardiac electrophysiologic study is necessary.

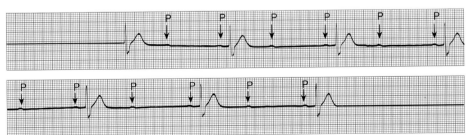

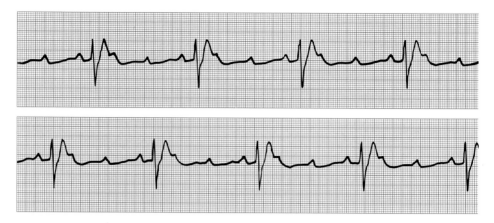

ECG 5-26. High-grade, or advanced, AV block. The P waves are regular and identical, with a rate of 107, but only every third P wave is conducted. Thus, this is still incomplete, or second-degree, AV block, but termed "high grade," or 3:1 (three P waves to each QRS complex). The anatomic site of block is below the AV node, similar to that of Mobitz II second-degree AV block.

ECG 5-27. Complete heart block with supraventricular escape rhythm. Regular, identical P waves with a normal P wave axis are seen at a rate of 105, consistent with sinus tachycardia. The QRS complexes are also regular, but at a rate of 44. With narrow QRS complexes, this implies a supraventricular (sinus, atrial, or AV nodal) origin of ventricular depolarization. It cannot be sinus or atrial, since the independent P wave rhythm occurring at a rate of 105 represents a sinus rhythm being conducted to and depolarizing the atrium. Thus, the rhythm driving the ventricles must be an AV nodal or junctional rhythm, confirmed by the rate of 44, consistent with the intrinsic rate of the AV node (40 to 55/minute).

Note that the P waves "march through" the QRS complexes: P_1 precedes a QRS complex by a reasonable time and, at first glance, might appear indeed to be responsible for a conducted QRS complex. However, P_2, P_4, and P_7 have no associated QRS complexes, and P_3 and P_5 have different and very long "PR intervals," the interval in the latter being so long that it is hard to believe that P_5 is truly responsible for the QRS that eventually follows.

P_6 is literally buried in the middle of a QRS complex, with the end of P_6 just poking out of the trailing edge of the QRS complex. Indeed, P_6 may not be recognized unless one plots the regular P wave rhythm with calipers, determines where P_6 *should* be, and then carefully inspects the QRS at that point and notes that it has a differently shaped trailing edge compared with all other QRS complexes. There is less downward S deflection, followed by an upward sharp notch, which is the buried P wave superimposed on the QRS. Clearly, P_6 has nothing to do with that QRS. P_1 and P_{10} just coincidentally happen to fall at a point where they could be related to a QRS, but it is obvious that the P wave rhythm everywhere is totally unrelated to the QRS rhythm, which is the definition of complete heart block.

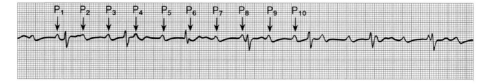

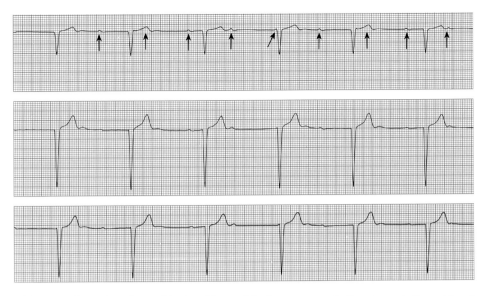

ECG 5-28. Complete heart block with ventricular escape rhythm in a rhythm strip of leads V_1, V_2 and V_3 only. The P waves (arrows) are regular and identical, with a normal P axis at rate 61, all consistent with normal sinus rhythm. The QRS complexes, however, are broad (0.12 second) and regular at a very slow rate, 36. A regular rhythm with broad QRS complexes and a rate of 36 is consistent with idioventricular rhythm; this patient has complete heart block below the AV node, either in the His bundle, in the bundle branches, or in all three fascicles. Thus, the only remaining source of ventricular depolarization is a site within the ventricles, or an idioventricular rhythm.

ECG 5-29. Atrial and ventricular premature contractions. Atrial premature contractions (APCs) occur before the next expected depolarization of the sinus. Note that the P wave of the APC (broken arrow) has a contour quite different from that of the P wave of sinus beats (best seen in lead II), since the APC originates at a different site and uses a different atrial pathway than a sinus beat. Both the sinus beat and the APC do spread through the ventricles via the AV node and the normal ventricular conduction system, so that the contour of the QRS is identical.

VPCs are seen in the precordial leads. Wide, bizarre QRS complexes without preceding P waves occur prematurely and are quite unlike the normal QRS complexes in any lead. The complex following the VPC in leads V_4, V_5 and V_6 is a junctional escape beat (JEB), occurring almost simultaneously with but probably unrelated to the P wave seen just peeking out of its leading edge.

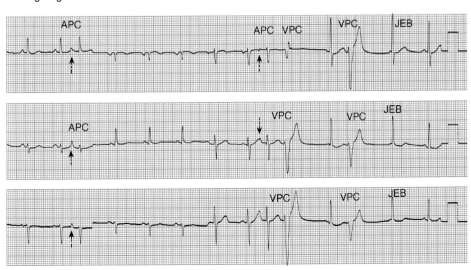

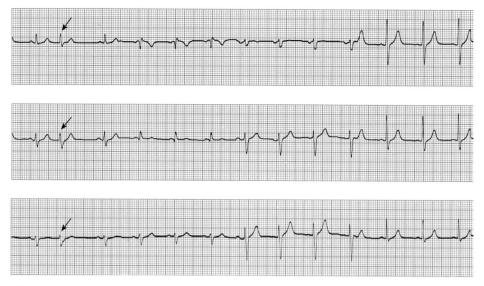

ECG 5-30. Junctional premature contraction (JPC). JPC (arrow) is quite similar to APC, except that no preceding P wave is seen. In some cases, there may be a P wave with a very short PR interval (analogous to a "high nodal" rhythm) or a P wave following the JPC (analogous to a "low nodal" rhythm).

ECG 5-31. Sinus pauses or sinus arrest, with junctional escape beats (JEB) in a two-channel ambulatory monitor strip. After the second and fifth beats, regular P waves pause for approximately 1.4 seconds, after which a narrow QRS complex without preceding P wave is seen (junctional escape beat). A narrow QRS complex without preceding P wave is of junctional origin; the intrinsic rate of the AV node or junction, 40 to 55/minute, corresponds to an interval of 1.50 to 1.09 seconds between depolarizations. Thus, if the sinus pauses are longer than the time needed to depolarize the AV node, the node will fire, capture the ventricles, and "escape" from the usual dominance of the sinus node.

Compare this ECG with 5-33, showing blocked APCs. When relatively short pauses are seen and the diagnosis of sinus pause is considered, a diligent search should be made for blocked APCs, which are a common cause of short pauses. This is particularly likely if conducted APCs are seen elsewhere in the tracing.

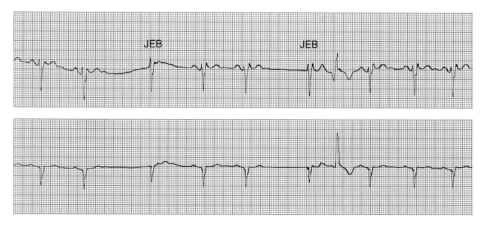

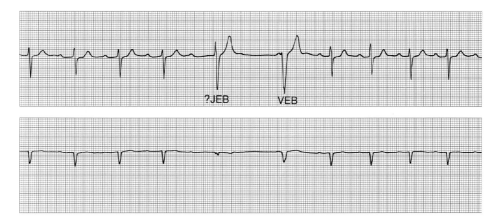

ECG 5-32. Sinus slowing and increasing AV block with two escape beats in a two-lead rhythm strip from a Holter monitor—recorded at 3 AM. The PR interval is quite long, 0.30 second in the first beat at left, and increases to 0.36 second in the third beat. The fourth P wave probably failed to conduct (Wenckebach second-degree AV block), and the fourth QRS complex is an escape beat occurring 1.16 seconds after the last conducted QRS. This may be a junctional escape beat (?JEB) or a ventricular escape beat. The sinus is probably reset by the JEB but fails to depolarize for 1.5 seconds, and the AV node, which would be expected to escape after 1.5 seconds at the latest (corresponding to an intrinsic junctional rate of at least 40/minute), also fails to fire.

Since neither the sinus nor the AV node depolarizes, a ventricular focus (intrinsic rate of idioventricular rhythm, 20 to 40/minute, corresponding to an interval of 3.0 to 1.5 seconds between depolarizations) is able to escape (the wide fifth QRS complex marked VEB for ventricular escape beat). The P wave occurring just at the leading edge of the VEB is too close to the VEB to be related to it, and is the sinus resuming normal activity. Worrisome as this whole sequence might appear at first glance, it is commonly seen in middle-of-the-night Holter recordings in people with little or no heart disease. It may all be a consequence of high vagal tone occurring during sleep.

ECG 5-33. Pauses due to blocked APCs. Although pauses following beats 3, 5, and 6 at first glance appear to be simply sinus pauses, note that the contour of the T waves at the solid arrows differs from that of most other T waves. The slightly more pointed shape is due to the P wave of the blocked APC, which occurs simultaneously with and slightly deforms the T wave. Since the APC has occurred soon after the prior QRS, the ventricle is still refractory and no QRS results. However, depolarization is transmitted backward to the sinus node, which "resets" and begins its process of automatic depolarization again, thus producing a short pause. When blocked P waves are hard to identify, the presumption that blocked APCs are the cause of pauses is greatly strengthened by finding definite conducted APCs elsewhere on the tracing, as in beat 10 of this example. Beat 10 is premature and is preceded by a P wave of unusual contour (deforming the preceding T wave) with a longer PR interval than occurs with most other beats on this rhythm strip, and the QRS is narrow — all characteristics of an APC.

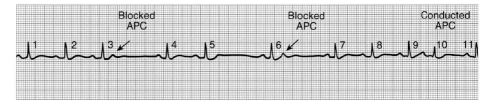

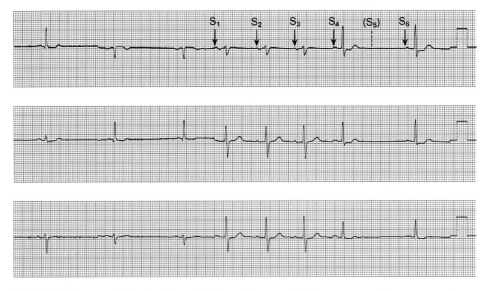

ECG 5-34. Sinus exit block. Although this tracing superficially appears to demonstrate a long sinus pause, precise measurement reveals that the interval from S4 (sinus node depolarization No. 4) to S6 is exactly double the interval from S3 to S4. As it is unlikely that a sinus pause would be exactly double the intrinsic SS interval of the sinus rhythm, one alternative explanation is that the sinus *is* actually depolarizing regularly all through the tracing but that the impulse *fails to exit* the sinus and depolarize the atrium at the point that should be S5 (broken line), and thus no P wave occurs. Remember that the sinus node, being a tiny structure, causes no discernible deflection on the standard ECG; thus, only electrophysiologic studies with intracardiac recording in close proximity to the sinus node could prove that the sinus actually continues to depolarize but its impulse is blocked on exiting.

ECG 6-1. Right atrial and right ventricular hypertrophy. This ECG demonstrates right axis deviation (QRS axis $+135°$); right atrial enlargement (P waves peaked and 3 mm tall in lead II, normal amplitude < 2.5 mm); and right ventricular hypertrophy (RVH), manifested by a tall R wave (actually an R′ wave) in lead V_1 (R′ wave $= 12$ mm, S wave essentially absent in lead V_1, normal R/S ratio < 1). A substantial S wave in leads V_5 and V_6 is also quite unusual and is a manifestation of RVH. An absolute R wave (or R′ wave) amplitude > 5 mm in lead V_1 or V_2 also signifies RVH according to some authorities. Note inverted T waves in leads V_1 and V_2. Compare with ECG 7-11, true posterior myocardial infarction.

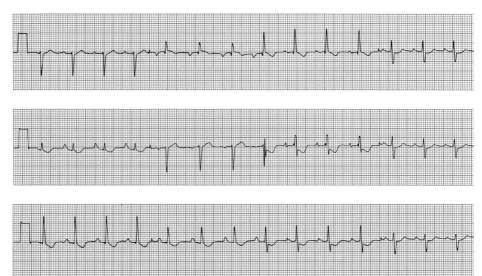

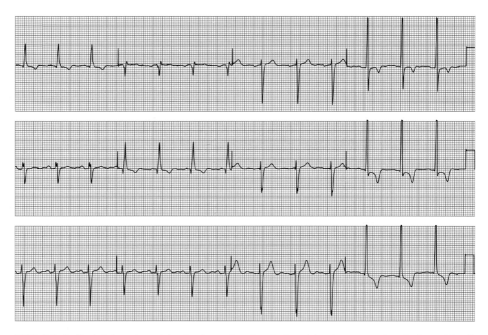

ECG 6-2. Left atrial and ventricular hypertrophy. Left atrial enlargement is manifested by P wave duration > 0.11 second (measured at 0.12 second in lead II or III), notching of the P wave with peaks separated by > 0.04 second (not seen in this tracing), and a negative P deflection in lead V_1 > 1.0 mm for > 0.04 second (borderline in this tracing). In addition, all the common criteria for left ventricular hypertrophy (LVH) are demonstrated in this ECG: R wave amplitude in lead I (11 mm) plus S wave amplitude in lead III (18 mm) equals 29 mm (normal < 25 mm); S wave in lead V_1 (20 mm) plus R wave in lead V_5 (>27 mm) equals at least 47 mm (normal < 35 mm); R wave in lead aVL equals 15 mm (normal < 11 mm). There are ST segment depressions and T wave inversions in leads I, aVL, V_4, V_5 and V_6, which are consistent with either myocardial ischemia or LVH; however, with the presence of all other criteria for LVH, it is highly likely that LVH is the cause.

ECG 6-3. Right bundle branch block (RBBB), left anterior hemiblock, and first-degree AV block ("trifascicular block"). Features of both RBBB and left anterior fascicular block are seen. RBBB causes a wide QRS (0.15 second), with the terminal portion of the QRS directed toward the right ventricle (rSR′ in lead V_1 and a terminal broad S wave in lead I). T wave inversions in right precordial leads (lead V_1 in this ECG) are normal with RBBB. This tracing also demonstrates marked left axis deviation (QRS axis = −71°, primarily negative QRS complex in leads II, III and aVF). This patient has block of both the right bundle branch and the left anterior fascicle of the left bundle; in addition, the greatly prolonged PR interval (0.39 second) is evidence of disease in the remaining avenue for AV conduction, the left posterior fascicle. Alternatively, there may be additional disease of the AV node itself.

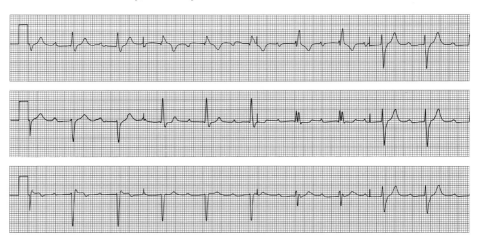

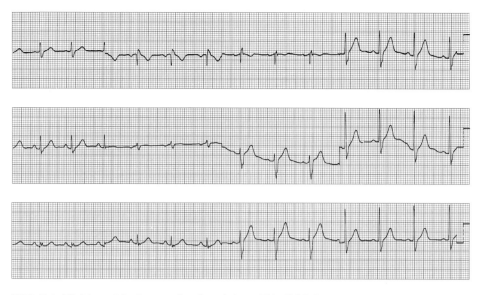

ECG 6-4. Right ventricular conduction defect. This ECG has a pattern similar to RBBB, with rSR' in lead V₁ and terminal S wave in leads I and V₆, but a QRS complex that is only slightly prolonged (0.10 second). (Normal QRS duration is < 0.09 second, definitely abnormal is > 0.12 second, and borderline 0.10 to 0.11 second.) Right ventricular conduction defect is a normal electrocardiographic variant and does not necessarily indicate any disease whatever.

ECG 6-5. Left bundle branch block (LBBB). The QRS is wide (0.13 second), with associated ST segment depressions, T wave inversions, and slowed upstroke of the initial portion of the QRS ("delayed intrinsicoid deflection") in leads reflecting primarily left ventricular forces, namely, leads I, aVL, V₅ and V₆. Very high QRS voltage is often seen (for example, leads V₁ through V₃), but this does not necessarily indicate ventricular hypertrophy since high voltage may result solely from the bundle branch block.

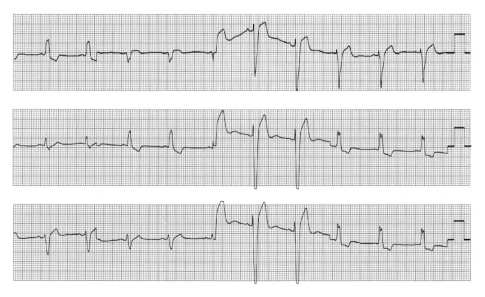

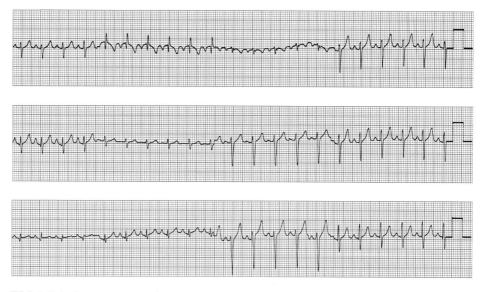

ECG 6-6. Left posterior fascicular block. The QRS is of normal duration (0.08 second), with rightward axis (QRS axis +174°) without RVH or anterolateral myocardial infarction.

ECG 6-7. Intraventricular conduction defect (IVCD). The QRS is wide (0.13 second), without features of RBBB (no rSR′ in lead V$_1$ or broad terminal S wave in lead I) or LBBB (no bizarre ST segment and T wave abnormalities or delayed QRS upstroke in left ventricular leads). Any wide (prolonged) QRS that cannot be diagnosed as one of the specific bundle branch blocks is given the generic name of IVCD.

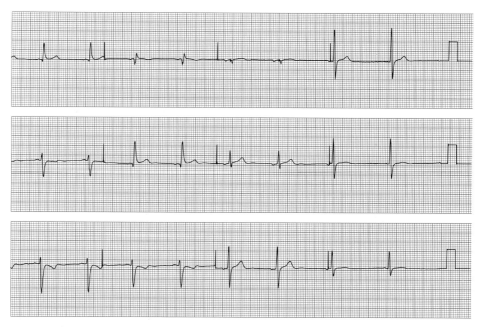

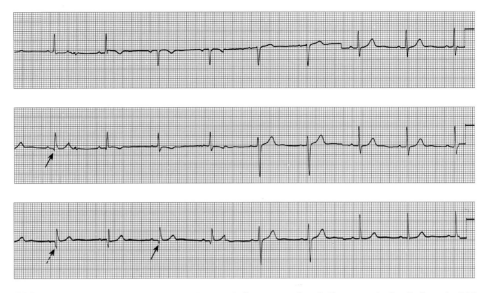

ECG 7-1. Normal ECG with normal septal Q waves. Small Q waves in leads II and aVF (arrows) are normal (about 0.02 second in duration and of small amplitude, much less than 25% of their respective R waves). A larger Q wave in lead III (broken arrow) may also be normal, and often disappears with change in heart orientation associated with deep inspiration. The lack of any inferior ST segment or T wave abnormalities further confirms that this is a normal ECG. Compare with Q waves of much greater duration (> 0.04 second) and amplitude (depth) in anterior (ECG 7-7) and diaphragmatic (ECGs 7-10 and 7-11) infarction.

ECG 7-2. Old, small anteroseptal myocardial infarction. Note the tiny Q waves at the onset of the QRS complex in leads V_2 and V_3 (arrows). Any Q wave, regardless of width or amplitude, is significant in leads V_2 and V_3 if these leads have the appearance of a lead positioned over the right ventricle or interventricular septum, that is, a smaller R wave and larger S wave. ST segment and T wave changes are often absent, making this type of infarction difficult to recognize.

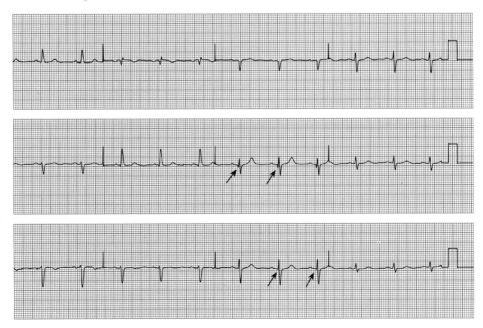

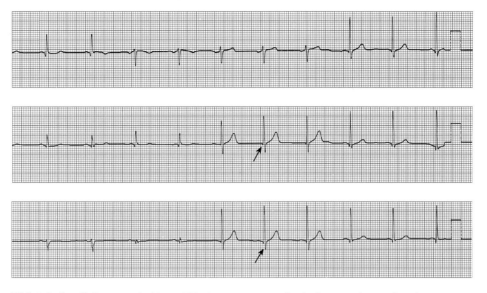

ECG 7-3. Small Q waves in V$_2$ and V$_3$ due to counterclockwise rotation, rather than anteroseptal myocardial infarction. Again, there are small Q waves in leads V$_2$ and V$_3$ (arrows). In this tracing, however, leads V$_2$ and V$_3$ have the appearance of a left precordial lead, that is, larger R wave and smaller or absent S wave. This is the result of either improper lead placement or rotation of the heart within the chest, so that the interventricular septum actually lies to the left of where it should be and electrodes in the usual V$_2$ and V$_3$ position are simply recording over the normal left ventricle, including a normal small septal Q wave.

ECG 7-4. Idiopathic hypertrophic subaortic stenosis (IHSS). Large Q waves are seen in leads II, III and aVF (arrows). The amplitude is greater than the R wave in lead III, equal to the R wave in lead aVF, and more than one-third of the R wave in lead II. Large Q waves are also seen in the precordial leads, with those in leads V$_2$ and V$_3$ being quite abnormal.

This ECG was recorded on a 72-year-old female with normal coronary arteries, no evidence of myocardial infarction, and a markedly hypertrophied and hypercontractile left ventricle at cardiac catheterization. She had a loud left sternal border systolic murmur, which increased with the Valsalva maneuver. All these findings confirm that the significant Q waves in this patient are caused by massive septal hypertrophy (due to IHSS) rather than by myocardial infarction.

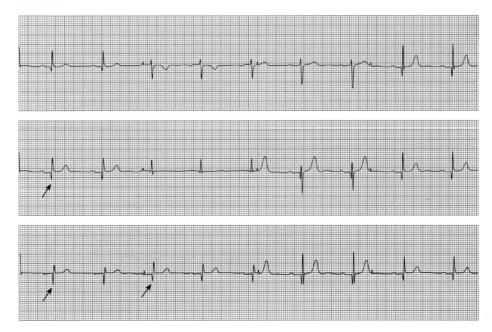

ECGs 7-5 through 7-7. Evolution of Acute Anterior Myocardial Infarction

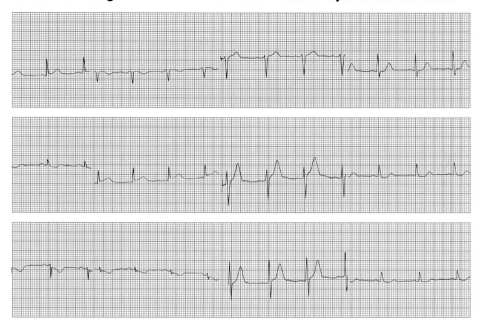

ECG 7-5. Acute anterior myocardial infarction 30 minutes after onset of symptoms. Subtle but definite ST elevation of approximately 1 mm in leads I, aVL and V_3 and a bit more in lead V_2, with peaked and rather full T waves in leads V_2 and V_3. R waves are still substantial in those leads, and T waves are upright.

ECG 7-6. Acute anterior myocardial infarction 6 hours after onset of symptoms. ST segment elevation is almost gone, and R wave amplitude in leads V_2 and V_3 has decreased considerably. T waves in leads V_2 through V_4 are inverted; T wave is low or biphasic in lead V_5.

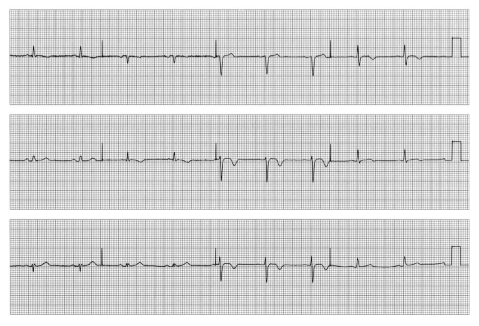

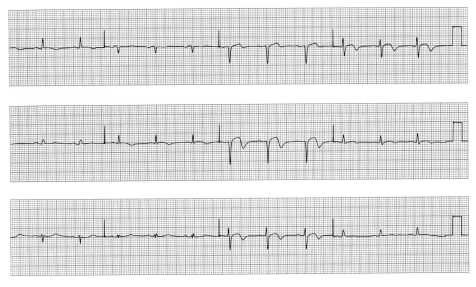

ECG 7-7. Anterior myocardial infarction 72 hours after onset of symptoms. The R wave has been completely lost, and QS complexes have developed in leads V_1 and V_2. T waves are now inverted in leads I, aVL and V_2 through V_5 and flat in lead V_6. The ST segments in leads V_1 and V_2 are elevated, which might indicate recurrent or continuing injury, but more likely (especially since the patient was pain-free at this time) suggests development of a ventricular aneurysm (the akinetic or dyskinetic area of infarcted myocardium). Such ST segment elevations may persist for months or even years.

ECG 7-8. Acute diaphragmatic infarction 1 hour after onset of symptoms. Marked ST segment elevation is seen in leads II, III and aVF. Subtle ST segment elevation in leads V_4 through V_6 probably represents lateral wall extension of what is likely a large infarction. The cause of the marked ST *depressions* in leads I, aVL, V_2 and V_3 is somewhat controversial. It may be "reciprocal," that is, simply the diaphragmatic current of injury reflected as ST depression instead of elevation on the opposite (anterior) wall, or it may represent additional ischemia or injury, probably on the posterolateral wall adjacent to the infarction. The rhythm is probably junctional with either AV dissociation or AV block. There are minuscule Q waves, but note that the R waves are still quite large in the diaphragmatic area of the acute infarction (leads II, III and aVF).

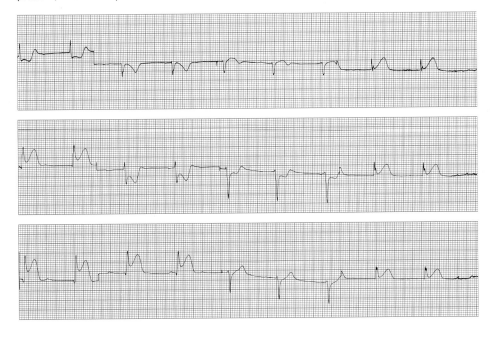

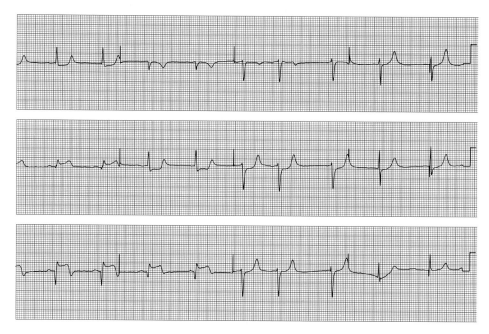

ECG 7-9. Acute diaphragmatic infarction 7 hours after onset of symptoms. ST segment elevations in leads II, III and aVF have diminished, and T waves have begun to invert. Most striking is the extraordinary loss of R wave in the short period (6 hours) since ECG 7-8. There are now significant Q waves in leads III and aVF. Sinus bradycardia has returned, with a probable APC in leads V_1, V_2 and V_3.

ECG 7-10. Old diaphragmatic myocardial infarction. Significant Q waves, indeed, total loss of R waves (the so-called QS complex) and T wave inversions in leads II, III and aVF are the end result of diaphragmatic (inferior) myocardial infarction that occurred many months ago. The very slight residual ST segment elevation may represent a ventricular aneurysm in the area of the infarction.

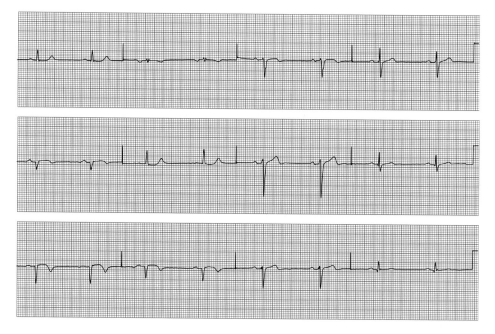

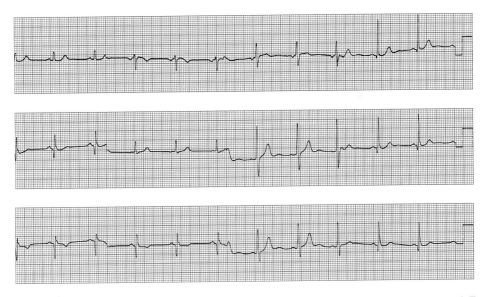

ECG 7-11. Old inferior and posterior myocardial infarction. Significant Q waves and T wave inversions in leads II, III and aVF signify diaphragmatic (inferior) infarction. However, in addition, the R wave in lead V_1 is tall (7 mm), exceeding the depth of the S wave in lead V_1 (only 5 mm). The T wave in lead V_1 is upright. Tall R wave (R>S) in lead V_1, with upright T wave, indicates true posterior myocardial infarction, not uncommon in the presence of inferior infarction. Neither right axis deviation nor right atrial enlargement is present. Compare with ECG 6-1, RVH, another situation in which R>S in lead V_1. However, RVH produces inverted T waves in lead V_1 and is associated frequently with right axis deviation and/or right atrial enlargement, neither of which is present in posterior myocardial infarction.

ECG 7-12. Counterclockwise rotation of the heart. This is another instance of tall R wave in lead V_1 (R wave amplitude 6 mm, exceeding S wave amplitude of 5 mm in lead V_1). In contradistinction to the two preceding ECGs, there are no signs of inferior myocardial infarction, right axis deviation, or right atrial enlargement. Indeed, lead V_1 simply appears the way a normal lead V_4 or V_5 would look. This is the result of marked counterclockwise rotation of the heart within the chest, so that the ECG electrode in the usual V_1 position is actually recording over the left ventricle, producing an R wave taller than the S wave. This is a common and benign situation and must not be confused with either true posterior myocardial infarction or RVH.

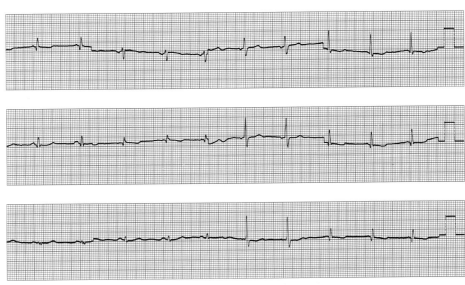

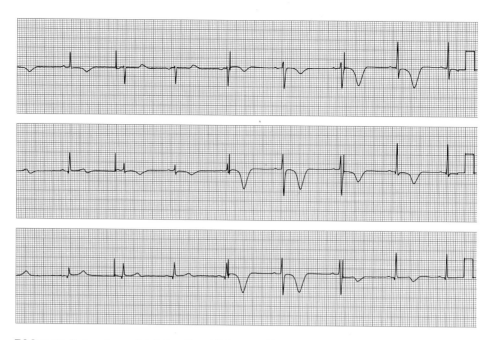

ECG 7-13. Subendocardial infarction. Widespread T wave inversions without any significant Q waves. Note that the electrocardiographic abnormalities are seen in anterior (leads I, V$_2$ through V$_4$), inferior (lead II), and lateral (leads aVL, V$_5$ and V$_6$) areas of the heart. The fact that abnormalities are not confined to the area of supply of any one or even two major coronary arteries is characteristic of widespread subendocardial infarction. The QT interval is also markedly prolonged (0.56 second, which is decidedly abnormal even at the slow heart rate of 50). QT prolongation is frequently caused by myocardial ischemia.

ECG 8-1. Acute pericarditis. ST segment elevations are seen in leads I, II, III, aVF and V$_2$ through V$_6$. The fact that the area of electrocardiographic abnormality does not correspond with the usual anatomic distribution of any one coronary artery suggests pericarditis, which might be confirmed by lack of Q waves, absence of serial electrocardiographic or serum enzyme changes of myocardial infarction, auscultation of a pericardial rub, or other clinical findings.

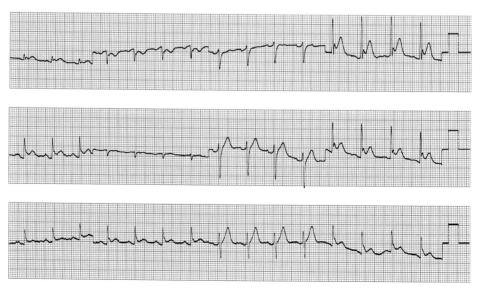

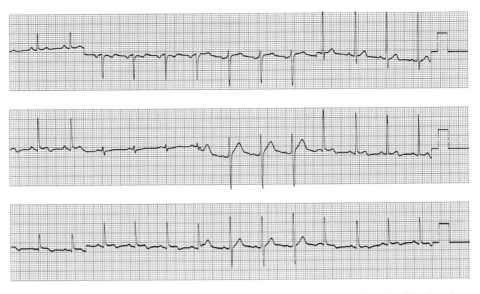

ECG 8-2. Chronic pericarditis. When acute pericarditis becomes chronic, ST elevations largely disappear, T waves usually become inverted in many leads, and voltage may decrease. (A major and sudden drop in voltage, not present in this ECG, may signify development of pericardial effusion.)

ECG 8-3. Early repolarization. Slight but definite ST segment elevations are seen in leads I, II, aVF and V_2 through V_6. When the patient is young (under 30 years of age) and has neither cardiac signs or symptoms nor other electrocardiographic abnormalities, early repolarization (a benign variant of the normal ECG) is the likely explanation for relatively minor ST elevations.

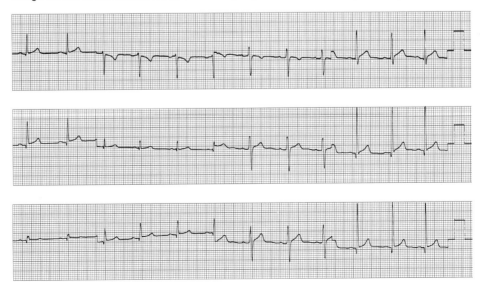

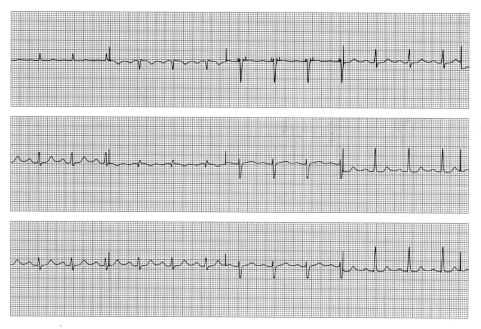

A

ECG 8-4A and B. ST segment depressions of myocardial ischemia. ECG 8-4A, the control tracing taken before exercise was begun, shows normal ST segments (at baseline with a heart rate of 80). ECG 8-4B was taken at 4 minutes of an exercise tolerance test, just as the test was stopped because of anginal pain, with a heart rate of 116. ST segment depression reaches 1.5 mm below the baseline at a point 0.08 second, or two small boxes, after the *end* of the QRS complex in leads V_5 and V_6; somewhat less ST segment depression is also seen in leads II, III and aVF. ST segment depressions are upsloping in leads II, III and aVF, horizontal in lead V_5, and downsloping (from left to right) in lead V_6, which increases the likelihood that they are caused by myocardial ischemia. This is a "positive" stress test.

B

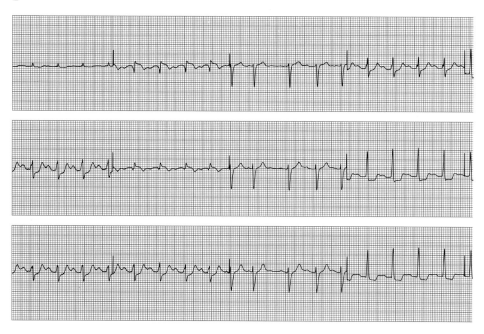

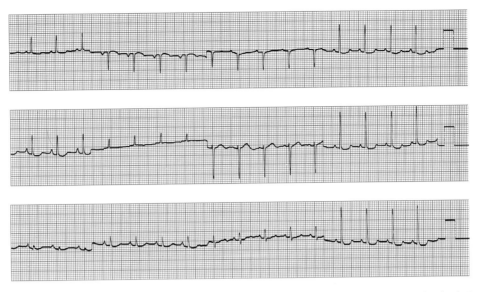

ECG 8-5. Nonspecific ST-T abnormalities. ST segments are depressed in many leads, but never more than 1 mm below baseline. The T wave vector is normal; that is, no specific area can be identified where ischemia or other myocardial abnormality might cause localized T wave inversions. (T waves tend to be inverted; that is, the T wave vector points *away* from an area where myocardial injury is localized.) Although T waves are not inverted on this ECG, they are of lower amplitude than normal (thus the designation "ST-T abnormalities").

ECG 8-6. Tall, peaked T waves. T waves in leads V_2 through V_4 at the upper limit of normal or above for adult T wave amplitude (see Table 2, page 76) are caused by hyperkalemia. See also ECGs 7-5 and 7-8, in which T waves are of substantial amplitude in the earliest stages of acute anterior and diaphragmatic infarctions. The tall T waves in those tracings may result from local hyperkalemia due to acute myocardial ischemia or injury.

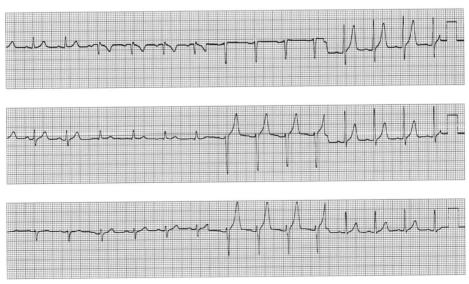

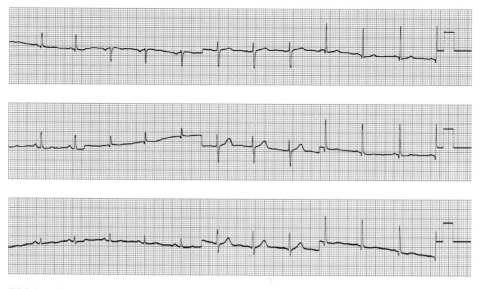

ECG 8-7. Flat T waves. T waves are flat and below the lower limit of normal for adults (Table 2) in most leads. This finding may be caused by a number of conditions, some serious and many relatively innocuous.

ECG 8-8. Widespread T wave abnormalities. T waves are flat (leads III and aVL), biphasic (lead V_6), or inverted (leads I, II, aVF and V_2 through V_5). These abnormalities were chronic in this patient, and not associated with any acute clinical events. Widespread T wave inversions tend to indicate myocardial disease, although the etiology (ischemia, hypertrophy, cardiomyopathy, among other causes) cannot be diagnosed from the ECG.

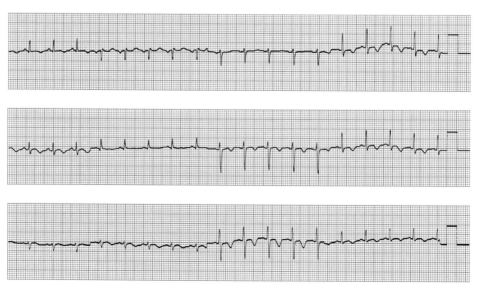

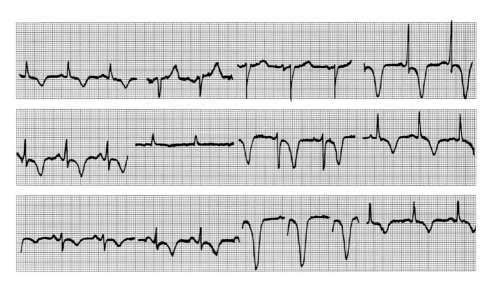

ECG 8-9. Cerebral T waves. This ECG shows a rare but striking example of an extracardiac cause of electrocardiographic abnormalities. These incredible deep and symmetric T wave inversions occurred in a young person with no known cardiac disease who had just had a major subarachnoid hemorrhage. The cardiac repolarization (T wave) abnormalities are presumably based on autonomic nervous system dysfunction.

ECG 8-10. Normal pediatric ECG. This ECG is from a normal 6-year-old child. In children, heart rates tend to be faster, PR intervals at the low end of normal (0.13 second here); and QRS durations also quite short, giving relatively narrow QRS complexes (0.08 second here). Right precordial T waves are *normally* inverted in leads V_1 through V_3 in babies and younger children and in leads V_1 and V_2 in older children, adolescents, and sometimes even young adults. T wave inversions in this ECG are seen in leads V_1, V_2 and V_3 and are normal at age 6.

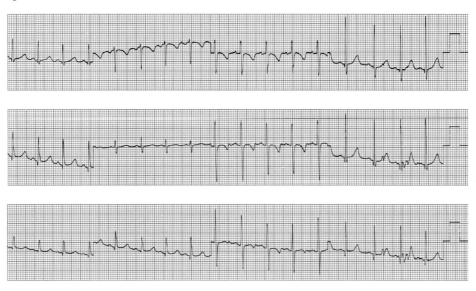

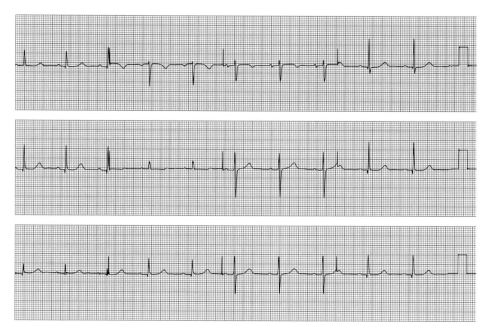

ECG 8-11. Prolonged QT interval. The QT interval measures 0.48 second, above the upper limit of normal for a female with a heart rate of 63 (see chart, Plate 7). Such QT prolongation has many causes, some serious and some benign.

ECG 8-12. Short QT interval. The QT interval measures 0.33 second, below the lower limit of normal for the heart rate of 70. The most common cause for this finding is hypercalcemia. The additional small wave after the T waves is termed a "U wave" (arrow). It is commonly associated with systemic hypertension and is of little clinical importance.

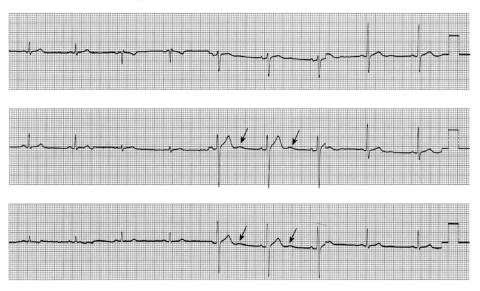